The Med Life Diet

12 Essential Steps to Creating Healthy Eating and Healthy Lifestyle Habits and Attitudes For Life !

Barbara Karafokas, MSc.

DEDICATION

I dedicate this book to my daughter who's got a beautiful smile and a wonderful sense of humour!

CONTENTS

The Med Life Diet

INTRODUCTION

Heart disease, cancer, Alzheimer's, diabetes and obesity are the leading causes of death today in the Western world.

A large number of us suffer from "minor" concerns such as being overweight, depression, high blood sugar, high blood pressure, indigestion, constipation, allergies, headaches and low energy to mention a few. Not many of us really experience good health and a zest for life.

Modern living has encouraged the most unhealthy lifestyle habits which lead to degenerative diseases.

Most of today's degenerative diseases are preventable, reversible and highly correlated to lifestyle habits.

As a matter of fact many people mistakenly think they're living healthy when they are doing the opposite. Anyone who wants to live a vibrant life, free of disease needs to be aware of what a healthy lifestyle truly is.

Whether your aim is to lose weight, reduce stress, detox, get fitter, eat better or just look great, 'The Med Life Diet', provides a realistic plan that sets you up for success.

In this book you will find all the information that you will need to create healthy eating and healthy lifestyle habits and attitudes for life !

Why 12 weeks?

Changing habits is hard, especially at first, requiring determination, discipline and dedication (the three D's) to make long lasting permanent changes. In this 12 week program, you will make changes slowly, adding in a new habit every week over the 12 week period.

This will give you adequate time to practice the new patterns and have them become a part of your life.

Book Structure

This book is divided into twelve weeks. It is designed to be studied in a linear fashion beginning from week one and ending at week twelve.

At the end of each chapter you will find a list of tasks for the week and where appropriate a meal plan and recipes.

 I am sure that it will bring about a positive change in your life

I look forward to helping you create a positive change and a healthier, vibrant life.

Let's Begin !

1 WEEK ONE

Changing … !

Change is an important part of life. The "I-Ching" or the Chinese book of change is based on the 'premise' that nothing ever remains the same.

What do I need to know in order to effect change? What do I need to learn in order to bring about change ?

These are questions we inevitably ask as we set out to create changes in our lives.

Some other powerful questions you can ask yourself are:

"What do I need to **unlearn** in order to prepare myself for a new and different way of thinking, feeling, doing, or being?"

Which bad habits do I have to release to take me closer to my goal ? Which behaviours do I consciously have to change to create positive changes in my life ?

Change and innovation both call for unlearning. To think anything new, and to see what could be new in things, you must learn to unlearn what you already know.

Think of experiences you've had of working towards change (in whatever respect), and reaching a moment in which you saw that change was actually possible, and more than possible, inevitable.

This is a moment of renewal – a new start. New beginnings always bring with them a world of new knowledge to be learnt.

"The only thing in life that is absolute is change" – Sophocles

Taking Responsibility for Your Life

There are some things that we can control and there are other aspects of our lives which we have no control of. How we treat our bodies and how we think and view life is in our control. If you desire to experience a higher level of health, there are some habits that you must incorporate into your life to enable you to experience that level of health and wellbeing which you wish to experience.

This Method Is Built On Self-Responsibility

The Western world is overweight or dying in increasing numbers from conditions linked with dietary and related lifestyle patterns. Heart disease, cancer, diabetes, kidney disease, and stroke – these are many of the killers of today.

The "minor" concerns we suffer from:

- Mood Swings
- Depression
- Tooth decay
- Indigestion
- Constipation
- Allergies
- Headaches
- Learning disabilities
- Hyperactivity
- Lethargy
- Skin disorders
- Weak nails and brittle hair
- Low libido

One of the basic problems is a fatal mix of dietary confusion with an increasingly inactive yet stressed lifestyle. Our diets and eating habits are highly imbalanced. Our stress levels are increasing, thereby undermining our ability to digest and utilize our foods properly. Our level of physical exercise is generally not enough to keep pace with what we eat and with the stresses we bear.

In some cases these imbalances exist because we lack information about nutrition, stress, and exercise; but the overall problem is more likely the result of changing lifestyle patterns and the choices that result from these.

With more people taking sedentary jobs, spending more hours in front of the TV, decreasing their exercise, obesity is on the rise.

Convenience and comfort are the main drivers of consumer food choices. We can now buy our fresh vegetables already peeled and cut up, and frozen dinners ready to pop into the microwave.

The increasing popularity of fast-food and restaurants has added to our diminishing control over our diets. Fast-foods are excessively high in the things we don't need – like salt, saturated and trans fats – and low in the things we do – like vitamins and minerals.

Food preferences are generally learned. With the use of modern advertising, food companies can stimulate our cravings, for snack foods and fast foods and teach our children that the only fun is had in eating saturated fats (potato crisps, French fries, and ice-cream), sugars (cookies, sweets and soft drinks), and high-protein "meals" (chicken nuggets, burgers and milkshakes).

The confusion around food shows up in the ways we have learned to use food to relieve emotional and physical pain.

To make things worse, to add to the issue of what we eat or don't eat in the way of nutrients, many of us are addicted to various drugs in foods, beverages, or food-like substitutes: sugar, caffeine, alcohol, nicotine, and a wide variety of pharmaceuticals.

It's a vicious circle in which each unbalancing factor leads to another and then turns back to reinforce itself. The more stressed you are, the more you may eat, the more pain you may create through increased weight or compounded guilt. The more pain you create, the more you may want to eat to ease it. Round and round it goes. Winning requires ending this cycle – moving into another circle altogether.

Tasks for This Week:

Start by going through your pantry and refrigerator to identify and discard common unhealthy foods.

1. Throw out all oils other than olive oil. If the olive oil smells old and rancid throw that out too and buy a fresh bottle.

2. Get rid of margarines, solid vegetable shortenings and products made with them such as biscuits, crackers and cakes. Also discard any products made with cottonseed oil.

3. Read the labels of all food products so that you can dispose of any containing partially hydrogenated oils of any kind.

4. Throw out any artificial sweeteners containing saccharin or aspartame and any products made with them.

5. Throw out any products containing artificial colouring (indicated on the label by phrases like "colour added", "artificially coloured", or the name of a particular dye, such as "FD&C red #3").

6. Make a commitment to read labels of all food products you buy. Pay special attention to the fat content, especially the saturated-fat content. I would like you to keep your total fat intake to about 20-25 percent of calories, and saturated-fat intake as low as possible. Do not buy products whose labels list more chemicals than recognizable ingredients.

7. Practice making healthier food choices based on the Healthy Food Guide.

Healthy Food Guide

A diet high in nutrients is the key to good health. Use the following as a guide when deciding which types of food to include in your diet and which ones to avoid in order to maintain good health.

Beans

Avoid: Canned pork and beans, canned beans with salt or preservatives, frozen beans.

Include: All beans cooked without animal fat or salt.

Beverages

Avoid: Alcoholic Drinks, coffee, sweetened milk chocolate, pasteurized and/ or sweetened juices and fruit drinks, sodas, tea (except herbal tea).

Include: Herbal teas, fresh vegetable juices and fresh fruit smoothies, cereal grain beverages (often sold as coffee substitutes), raw cacao, dark chocolate powder, mineral or distilled. Nut and seed milks. E.g. almond milk.

Dairy Products

Avoid: All soft Cheeses made from cow's milk, all pasteurized or artificially coloured cheese products and ice-creams.

Include: Goat cheeses, cottage cheese, unsweetened yoghurt, kefir (airani), goat's milk, yoghurt, cheese such as Feta cheese, Halloumi cheese, whey cheeses (E.g. Ricotta, Brunost, Anari, Xynomizithra, Anthotyros, Manouri).

Eggs

Avoid: Fried or pickled

Include: Boiled, poached, omelet, scrambled (limit of four

14

weekly). Preferably organic or free range.

Fish

Avoid: All fried fish, salted fish, anchovies, herring, fish canned in oil. Tuna not more than once every 2 wks as it contains high levels of mercury.

Include: All freshwater white fish, salmon, broiled or baked fish, water packed sardines. Albacore tuna as it has lower levels of mercury.

Fruits

Avoid: Canned, bottled or frozen fruits with sweeteners added, oranges.

Include: All fresh, frozen, stewed, or dried fruits without sweeteners (except oranges in moderation as they can be highly allergenic and are acidic to the stomach and may cause acid reflux), unsulfured fruits, home-canned fruits. Preferably organic.

Grains

Avoid: All white flour products, white rice, pasta, crackers, cold cereals, instant types of oatmeal and other hot cereals.

Include: All whole grains and products containing whole grains: cereals, breads, muffins, whole-grain crackers, cream of wheat or rye cereal, buckwheat, millet, oats, brown rice, quinoa, amaranth, wild rice. (limit yeast breads to three servings per week). Sourdough bread is a better option.

Meats

Avoid: Red Meats, fatty meats (e.g. beef, lamb, pork), all forms of pork, hot dogs, luncheon meats, smoked, pickled, and processed meats, corned beef, duck, goose, spare ribs, gravies, organ meats.

Include: Preferably skinless Turkey & chicken, game meat. Red meats and liver to be eaten in moderation (1 per week). Choose grass fed, organic meats or game.

Nuts and Seeds

Avoid: All salted or roasted nuts, peanuts.

Include: All fresh raw nuts and seeds such as: almonds, walnuts, hazelnuts, cashews, pecans, Brazil, sunflower seeds, pumpkin seeds, flaxseeds, sesame seeds. (peanuts in moderation as they contain aflatoxin a mold which causes liver cancer).

Oils (fats)

Avoid: All saturated fats, hydrogenated margarine, refined processed oils, shortenings, hardened oils.

Include: All cold-pressed oils such as olive, walnut, flaxseed, coconut and sesame oil. Only cook with olive and sesame oil.

Seasonings

Avoid: Black or white pepper, salt, hot red peppers, all types of vinegar except pure natural apple cider vinegar.

Include: Garlic, onions, cayenne, all herbs, dried vegetables, apple cider vinegar, tamari, miso, seaweed, dulse.

Soups

Avoid: Canned soups made with salt, preservatives, MSG (monosodium glutamate), or fat stock, all creamed soups with fresh cream.

Include: Homemade (salt- and fat-free) bean, lentil, pea, vegetable, barley, brown rice, onion.

Sprouts

Avoid: All seeds cooked in oil or salt.

Include: Sprouts raw or slightly cooked, wheatgrass, all raw seeds. Avoid all Kidney Bean sprouts - they are extremely poisonous.

Sweets

Avoid: White, brown, or raw cane sugar, corn syrups, chocolate, sugar candy, fructose (except that in fresh whole fruit), all syrups (except pure maple syrup), all sugar substitutes, jams and jellies made with sugar.

Include: Barley malt or rice syrup, small amounts of raw unprocessed honey, maple syrup, stevia, date syrup, unsulfured blackstrap molasses.

Vegetables

Avoid: All canned or frozen with salt additives

Include: All raw, fresh, frozen (no additives). Preferably undercook most vegetables from 1 – 4 minutes by stir frying, steaming or grilling. Oven baked are also nutritious.

2 WEEK TWO

Vibrant Fruit Meals

Fruit

Fruits are considered nature's perfect foods with many positive qualities. They are delicious, healthy, juicy with a high water content similar to that of the human body.

Fruits are also well stocked in nutrients, particularly important vitamins as A and C, a little of the B's, and E in seeds. Many minerals, such as calcium, magnesium, copper, a little iron, manganese and other trace minerals, are also present in fruits, especially when they are contained in the water and soil that nourishes the plants or trees.

They are low in calories, fat, sodium and high in fiber an additional benefit in our commonly high-fat, high salt and low-fiber culture.

Fruits are cleansing and detoxifying easy to digest and utilize and so they usually have a low allergenic potential (allergy comes mainly from the protein components of food).

Occasionally, someone is sensitive to such fruits as oranges or tomatoes, but this is less common than with other regularly used foods, such as milk, wheat, and other grains.

Fruits may have a cooling and calming action for the body and nervous system and may be helpful in reducing body stress. This is due to the natural nutrient content. Fruit consumption may help strengthen our immune system as well.

It is most natural and economical to eat fruits fresh in season. It is ideal to wash them to clean off any sprays, germs, and environmental contaminants and to eat organic fruits whenever possible.

Eating fruit in its ripe state is probably best for our body, as the "green" or unripe fruits may be more irritating.

Fresh fruit is best from a nutritional standpoint. Fresh frozen is next, as the fruits lose very little of their nutrients, and then dried fruit.

Add in a fruit meal a day. Fruit should be eaten on an empty stomach and preferably in the morning.

The three main ways which you may eat fruit are:

1) Fruit Smoothie
2) Fruit Salad
3) Whole fruit, e.g. an apple, a banana

Health Tip:

It is best to add some protein or fat to the fruit meal. This slows down blood sugar absorption, which ensures a healthier effect on the body.

E.g. RAW : Flax seeds, chia seeds, cacao nibs, sesame seeds, sunflower seeds, pumpkin seeds, almonds, walnuts, hazelnuts, pistachios, a tablespoon of goat's or sheep's yoghurt, tahini, flaxseed oil, coconut oil.

Health food shops have wonderful 'Omega 3' sprinkle mixes which may be added to fruit salads.

Smoothie Tips:

The basic formula for a smoothie is 1 cup of liquid such as water, fruit juice, goat's milk, rice milk, almond milk, oat milk, or other nut milks. Add 1 cup of fruit, either fresh or frozen, and you have your base drink.

Smoothies are so rich and creamy that you can hide ingredients such as ground flaxseed, wheat germ, flaxseed oil, coconut oil, sheep or goat's yoghurt, tahini.

On top of that you can make it more nutritious by adding wholefood supplements such as probiotics, algae (spirulina, chlorella), aloe vera, bee pollen, vitamin C, and many others without changing the flavour too much.

Drink your smoothies as soon as possible after making them so the ingredients are fresh and have not oxidized. If you do have to take them with you to work, put them in a dark, airtight container such as a thermos and add in a couple of ice cubes.

A Smoothie Secret:

Frozen fruit makes thicker smoothies. Chop up some fruit, place in a container and store in the freezer. Bananas, strawberries, grapes, peaches, cherries and blackberries are always handy to have frozen.

Tasks for This Week:

1. Start your day with lemon water. Lemon water boosts your immune system, stimulates the liver to release toxins, balances PH and reduces your body's overall acidity, helps with weight loss, aids digestion, is a diuretic, clears the skin, freshens breath, relieves respiratory problems and helps to kick the coffee habit by reducing cravings, rich in vitamin C and also cleanses the liver.

2. Lemon water is then followed by a **fruit meal** and a healthy Mediterranean breakfast meal. A space of at least 30 minutes must be left between your fruit meal and Mediterranean breakfast.

Fruit Meal Recipes

Fruit Salads and Muesli's

Barbara's Nutty Breakfast

1   apple chopped
1   banana sliced
2   tbs goat's/sheep's yoghurt OR 1 tbs tahini (for Vegans)
2   tbs crushed walnuts
1   tbs ground flaxseeds
1   tbs chia seeds
1   tbs goji berries
1   tsp cacao nibs
1   tsp coconut oil
½   tsp raw unpasteurized honey (optional)
½   tsp sprinkle of cinnamon

Place chopped fruit in a bowl. Add all other toppings sprinkle with cinnamon, drizzle with honey and enjoy !

Note: You may find mixed seed packets at health food shops which definitely speeds up the preparation process. You can add other sprinkles like sesame seeds, chia seeds, cacao nibs.

Raw Muesli

2 -4 tbs breakfast oats soaked overnight in a little spring water.
1   grated apple (pear or banana)
½   cup low fat yoghurt (sheep or goat's yoghurt)

Mix all the ingredients and sprinkle with toasted seeds or mixed nuts.

Muesli

½   cup muesli (without added sugar)
1   banana chopped (OR 1 apple OR a pear)
1- 2 tbs goat's or sheep's yoghurt
1   tsp raw unpasteurized honey

Place muesli in a bowl. Add chopped banana (or fruit of your choice), then add yoghurt and drizzle with honey.

Easy Oat Breakfast

2-3 tbs oats
1   tbs sunflower seeds or other nuts or seeds (e.g. crushed
        walnuts, almonds)
1   tbs raisins or goji berries or blackcurrants
½   cup almond milk or water either hot or cold
¼   tsp cinnamon
½   tsp raw unpasteurized honey

Place oats, sunflower seeds and raisins in a bowl. Add water or almond milk. Sprinkle with cinnamon and honey.

Fruit Salad with Cinnamon Raisin Sauce

Dice into bite sized pieces and place in large bowl:

4 apples
2 pints strawberries
3 pears
4 sliced bananas
2 peaches / nectarine, etc (whatever is in season)

In Blender:
½ cup raisins
1 cup shredded coconut

2-4 oranges or mandarins juiced
1 tsp cinnamon
1 tbs ginger
1 tsp allspice
1 tsp clove

Blend for 30 seconds so that it is still a little chunky. Pour sauce over fruit salad and toss well. Garnish with more shredded coconut.

Mixed Melon Salad

1 small watermelon
1 cantaloupe
1 honeydew melon

Scoop out balls. Drizzle with honey acacia honey and decorate with flowers and mint leaves.

Banana Coconut Salad

6   bananas – sliced
1   pint strawberries or other berries
¼ cup flaked unsweetened coconut
½ cup chopped walnuts (soaked 8 hours)
½ cup fresh squeezed orange juice or mandarin juice

Combine and serve.

Basic Quick and Simple Fruit Meal

- Chop up any combination of two fruits which are in season.
- Add a tablespoon of various RAW nuts and seeds such as: sesame seeds, flaxseeds, walnuts, almonds, hazelnuts, tahini or goat's / sheep's yoghurt.
- Add in a tablespoon or two of dried fruit such as raisins, black currants, figs, dates, apricots.
- Sprinkle with spices such as cinnamon, nutmeg or cloves.

Variation: In winter: You may warm up some almond milk and pour it over the top or lightly cook apples or pears.

Smoothies

Nut Milks

1 cup any nuts or seeds, soaked overnight
1 tbs raw, unprocessed honey or maple syrup
    (optional, I like mine without a sweetener)
1 tsp Celtic salt or Himalayan Pink salt (optional)
3 cups water

Thoroughly blend all ingredients in a blender until smooth. Strain mixture through a cheese cloth bag. Pour into a jar.

Energy Boost Banana Shake

Bananas provide electrolytes and easily absorbed calories to boost energy.

1 cup alternative milk. (rice, almond, sesame etc...)
1 banana (fresh or frozen)

Add protein powder, or other supplements or superfoods such as bee pollen, royal jelly, aloe vera, flax seed oil, green powder (such as spirulina, chlorella, wheat grass, barley grass)

Blend all ingredients in a blender until smooth and drink immediately.

Refreshing Berry Cooler

Berries contain cleansing fiber and antioxidants.

1   cup alternative milk or juice (e.g. orange)
½ - 1 cup berries (fresh or frozen)
1-2   tbs protein powder, superfood or other supplement
1   banana

Blend all ingredients in a blender until smooth and drink immediately.

Cherry Vanilla

1   cup water
½ cup goat's yoghurt
¼ stick vanilla or a drop vanilla essence
1 ½ cups frozen pitted cherries, or other berries in season

Blend all ingredients in a blender until smooth and drink immediately.

Icy Pineapple

1   orange
1   cup frozen pineapple chunks
½ frozen very ripe medium banana
¼ lemon with peel
1   glass water

Blend all ingredients in a blender until smooth and drink immediately.

Avocado Citrus Smoothie

1   small avocado
1   small orange, peeled
½ small grapefruit
¼ lemon with peel
2   handfuls goji berries, soaked for an hour or so
1   cm cube ginger
1   cup water

Blend all ingredients in a blender until smooth and drink immediately.

Carob's Delight

1   glass almond milk or water
1   banana (frozen or fresh)
1-2 soft pitted dates (soak in water overnight)
1-2 tbs carob powder (depending on how chocolaty
     you want it)
¼ tsp cinnamon powder
¼ cloves powder

Blend all ingredients in a blender until smooth and drink immediately.

Oat, Banana & Pear Smoothie

1   medium banana
1   medium pear, very soft and ripe
1   cup almond milk
¼ cup oats
¼ tsp cloves or mixed spices
1   tsp raw, unprocessed honey

Blend all ingredients in a blender until smooth and drink immediately. This smoothie is very filling.

Mango and Peach Smoothie

1 mango
3 peaches
3 tbs low-fat yoghurt or 2 tbsp tahini
1 glass water

Stone the mango and the peaches and cut both fruits into chunks. Blend all ingredients in a blender until smooth and drink immediately.

Banana & Peach Smoothie with Strawberries

1 banana
1 peach
12 strawberries
3 tbs low-fat yogurt

Peel the banana and break it up into chunks. Remove the stone from the peach and chop it into chunks. Remove the green stalks from the strawberries. Put all the ingredients into the blender and blend until smooth.

Savory Green Smoothies

Green smoothies are great for afternoons when you may need an energy boost. You may also have them late mornings if you wish, depending on your mood.

Italiano smoothie

6   leaves of red leaf lettuce
¼   bunch of fresh basil
½   lime juiced
½   red onion
2   celery sticks
¼   avocado
2   cups water

Blend well and drink.

Tomato Smoothie

5   ripe tomatoes
¼   bunch parsley
2   cucumbers
1   lemon, juiced
1   clove, garlic   (optional)
1   tbs olive oil
¼   tsp turmeric
1   cup water
    pinch cayenne pepper

Blend and drink.

Green Med Shake

2 ½   cups spinach
½   bunch fresh coriander
1   clove garlic
½   red bell pepper
½   lemon, juiced
1   tsp honey.

3   Roma tomatoes
2   cups water

Blend and Drink.

Delicious Green

5   leaves spinach
2   tomatoes
1   cm cube ginger
2   cups water
½   lemon juice
¼   avocado
¼   tsp pink himalayan salt

Blend and drink.

Smoothie Secrets

❖   Frozen fruit makes thicker smoothies. Peel overripe bananas and other fruit such as strawberries and grapes and keep them in the freezer. Preferably store them in a glass container with a plastic lid.

Morning Meal Plan

Monday
First Thing in the Morning
1 glass room temperature, lemon water, add juice of ¼ - ½ lemon

Breakfast
Barbara's Nutty Breakfast

Mid-Morning Snack
2 thin slices anari (low fat whey cheese),
drizzle with 1 tsp honey or 1 tbs carob syrup

OR savoury version

2 thin slices anari cheese
1 tomato
1 cucumber
Drizzle 1/2 tsp olive oil and sprinkle with salt, pepper and oregano

20 Minutes before Lunch
Drink one or two glasses of water or herbal tea

Tuesday
First Thing in the Morning
1 glass room temperature, lemon water, add juice of ¼ - ½ lemon

Breakfast
1 glass Energy Boost Banana Shake

Mid-Morning Snack
1/2 cup sugar-free muesli
1 tbs of goat's / sheep's yoghurt
1/2 tsp honey

20 Minutes before Lunch
Drink one or two glasses of water or herbal tea.

Wednesday
First Thing in the Morning
1 glass room temperature, lemon water, add juice of ¼ - ½ lemon

Breakfast
1 bowl Banana, Coconut Salad

Mid-Morning Snack
1 boiled egg
1 slice barley, rye or whole grain brown bread
1 tsp butter or mayonnaise or olive oil to spread on bread (optional)
1 cucumber, sliced
1 tomato, sliced
3 olives

20 Minutes before Lunch
Drink one or two glasses of water or herbal tea

Thursday
First Thing in the Morning
1 glass room temperature, lemon water, add juice of ¼ - ½ lemon

Breakfast
1 large glass Carob's Delight Smoothie

Mid-Morning Snack
Easy Oat Breakfast

20 Minutes before Lunch
Drink one or two glasses of water or herbal tea

Friday
First Thing in the Morning
1 glass room temperature, lemon water, add juice of ¼ - ½ lemon

Breakfast
1-2 pieces of fruit of your choice e.g. 1 peach and 1 apple

Mid-Morning Snack
1 bowl Raw Muesli

20 Minutes before Lunch
Drink one or two glasses of water or herbal tea

Saturday
First Thing in the Morning
1 glass room temperature, lemon water, add juice of ¼ - ½ lemon

Breakfast
1 glass Oat, Banana and Pear smoothie

Mid-Morning Snack
2 thin slices goat's cheese like feta or halloumi or anari
1 slice barley, rye or whole grain brown bread
1 cucumber, sliced
1 tomato, sliced
1 tsp olive oil or butter
Sprinkle oregano, salt and pepper

20 Minutes before Lunch
Drink one or two glasses of water or herbal tea.

Sunday
First Thing in the Morning
1 glass room temperature, lemon water, add juice of ¼ - ½ lemon

Breakfast
1-2 pieces of fruit of your choice e.g. 1 peach and 1 apple

Mid-Morning Snack
Omelet with 2 -3 eggs and vegetables of your choice like mushrooms, spinach, asparagus, onions, peppers etc.
1 tbs grated goat's cheese
Serve with cucumber, tomato slices and olives.

20 Minutes before Lunch

Drink one or two glasses of water or herbal tea.

Anari is a fresh mild whey cheese produced in Cyprus.
It is a by-product of Cypriot traditional cheese called halloumi and
other cheese products. Anari is favoured as a breakfast cheese as it is
an easily digestible low-fat cheese with a bland flavour. The unsalted
anari is eaten for breakfast. Salted anari is dried, grated and
sprinkled over pasta.

Anari cheese may be substituted with similar cheeses such as
mizithra cheese, cottage cheese, ricotta cheese, Brunost,
Xynomizithra, Anthotyros, Manouri or other low fat unsalted goat's
cheeses.

3 WEEK THREE

Scrumptious Greens !

Vegetables

The Latin word for vegetables means "to enliven or animate".
Most vegetables are very high in water and necessary vitamins and
minerals and low in fat and protein. A wide variety of vegetables are
predominantly carbohydrate, with important fiber bulk.

Vitamins C and A, potassium, calcium, magnesium, and iron are the
most commonly rich nutrients, along with some B vitamins and
other trace minerals.

The dark leafy greens, yellow or orange vegetables, such as squash
and carrots, and red ones such as peppers are high in beta-carotene,
which produces vitamin A in our body.

Many of the nutrients may be partially lost when cooking vegetables.
Vitamin C and some minerals may dissolve in the water, and the B
vitamins may be destroyed by heat and also lost in the water, yet
overall, the basic nutrition and fiber will still remain.

The flavours, many colours, and varieties of textures of vegetables
are a distinct advantage to those who enjoy natural tastes and
aesthetic eating. However, the low salt and fat content tends to
reduce interest for people who have developed a taste for those
attractions.

Quite often, children refuse, often passionately, from the pleasures of
vegetables, as their tastes may tend toward sweet flavours and they
may oppose the often slightly bitter flavours of greenery.

The chlorophyll that is part of most plants, especially high in the
green vegetables, has special properties. It is the basic component of
the plant's blood, just as hemoglobin is in ours. Instead of iron as the
focal part, as it is with our blood, magnesium is the center of the

chlorophyll molecule, and thus many plants have a good level of magnesium.

Chlorophyll is produced as a result of the sun's effects on the plants, and it is known to have revitalizing and refreshing effects when used in humans.

Here are just a few benefits you may experience as chlorophyll…

- Aids your body in processing more oxygen
- Cleanses key elimination systems like your bowel, liver, and blood
- Helps purify your blood and clear away toxins
- Normalises blood pressure
- Supports elimination of molds in your body
- Helps neutralize bad air you might breathe in
- Promotes growth and repair of your tissues
- Provides intestinal nourishment and has a soothing or healing effect on the mucous linings
- Used beneficially for skin ulcers
- Chlorophyll can help prevent cancer and is being used in cancer therapy

Because of their beta-carotene and selenium levels, vegetables are thought to help reduce cancer rates.

The cruciferous family vegetables, such as broccoli, Brussels sprouts and cauliflower, have a further anticancer effect, though the exact mechanism has not yet been determined.

Health Tip:

To obtain the complete health benefits of vegetables, the best way to eat most of them is in their raw form. Lightly steaming them for about two minutes or until they turn a very bright green is also ideal. Quickly remove them from the hot water and serve immediately. To stop the cooking process you may also rinse them in cold water and then consume them at a later time at your convenience.

Seasonal Eating Of Fresh Foods

One of the most natural concepts of eating is that of consuming primarily foods that are grown in the area in which we live, and consuming them near the time when they are grown.

Eating seasonally keeps us aligned to the Earth, its elements, and the cycles of nature. Eating seasonally is also a most economical dietary pattern and gives us potentially the cleanest foods, as fewer chemicals are needed to store or ship them.

Another important reason to eat this way is that the right type of fuel is provided to protect you from the weather. The environment provides the best foods to support our health and keep us in balance.

For example, in summer's hottest months, the juiciest of fruits are available. Fruits and fruit juices help to cool the body. In winter, when it is cold and wet, foods that require most cooking are the most common.

Guide to Seasonal Vegetables

Spring

Artichoke, asparagus, beets, beet greens, bok choy, broccoli, Brussels' sprouts, cabbage, cauliflower, carrot, celery, chard, chickweed, chicory, coriander, collard greens, dandelion greens, garlic, onions, peas, leeks, lettuce all types, mint, mushrooms, mustard greens, nettle, parsley, radish, spinach.

Summer

Artichoke, beet and beet greens, bell pepper, cabbage, carrots, celery, chili pepper, chive, corn, cucumber, eggplant, green beans, peas, lettuce, new potatoes, okra, onion, parsley, radish, rhubarb, spinach, yellow squash, crookneck, scallop and zucchini, peas, tomato and watercress.

Autumn

Bell pepper, broccoli, burdock root, cabbage, red, green, carrot, cauliflower, corn, cucumber, eggplant, garlic (dried), horseradish, Jerusalem artichoke, leeks, lettuces, okra, onions, parsnips, potatoes, pumpkin, rutabaga, shallot, spinach, squash (hard) different varieties, squash (soft) different varieties, string beans, tomato, turnip.

Winter

Bok Choy, Broccoli, Brussels' sprouts, burdock root, butternut squash, cabbages, carrots, cauliflower, chard, collard greens, garlic, Jerusalem artichoke, leeks, onions, parsnip, potatoes, rutabaga, seaweeds (e.g. dulse, kelp), spinach.

Tasks for This Week:

1. Add in a fresh, raw salad meal a day. For the adventurous add in a fresh vegetable juice to your health regime about 3 - 4 times a week or more.

2. Salad should make up 4/5 of your plate. The remaining 1/5 is made up of toppings.

Below are some toppings you may choose from:

Tuna
Sardines
Beans, chick peas, lentils, (other pulses)
Prawns
Shrimps
Mussels
Goat's cheeses, such as feta, halloumi, chevre, unsalted anari,
Cottage cheese
Sheep's or goat's yoghurt
Raw nuts and seeds (almonds, walnuts, sunflower seeds, sesame seeds, pumpkin seeds, pine nuts, pistachios, hazelnuts, brazil nuts, pecan nuts)
Olives
Capers
Tahini
Humus
Tarama
Avocado
Boiled Eggs
Steamed vegetables (artichokes, green beans, sweet corn, peas, asparagus, boiled potato)
Sprouts (lentil, chick peas, mung bean, watercress, sunflower)

These are just some suggestions, please feel free to use your imagination and create your own, healthy delicious salads !

Salad Meal Recipes

Salad Tip:

 The principles of making nutritious salads are quite simple.

Mix together these three types of vegetables. One root, one bulb (or fruit) vegetable, and one leaf vegetable. Sprinkle with fresh or dried herbs and add a delicious and nutritious dressing.

Root Vegetables: carrots, celeriac, turnips, onions, leeks, beetroot, radishes, white radishes, etc.

Bulb or 'fruit' vegetables: tomatoes, red and green peppers, fennel, avocado, cucumber, cauliflower, celery, broccoli, zucchinis, mushrooms, Calabrese, etc.

Leaf Vegetables: lettuce, young dandelion leaves, young beet tops, red or white cabbage, Brussels sprouts, spring onions, spring greens, spinach, chicory, endive, etc. Watercress, cress and sprouted grains and seeds can be used in any combination, or on their own, or as a garnish.

To increase a salad's protein content you can sprinkle it with three-seed mixture, an excellent source of both omega-3 and omega-6 essential fatty acids.

Mix together equal quantities of sunflower, pumpkin and sesame seeds, grind in a coffee grinder, then sprinkle on the salad. Three-seed mixture can also be added to breakfasts and to drinks. Once ground it should be stored in the refrigerator.

You can also give salads a protein lift with mixed nuts, or sprouted seeds or grains, or add some soft goat's cheese, free-range chicken, chopped boiled eggs, prawns, fish, etc.

Cucumber Tomato Salad

1 medium cucumber
3 ripe tomatoes
1 tbs cold pressed olive oil
1 tbs apple cider vinegar or lemon juice
Pinch coarse sea salt
Pinch oregano

Chop washed and cleaned cucumber and tomatoes in a bowl. Drizzle olive oil and sprinkle with salt and oregano

Village Salad

4   tomatoes
1   cucumber
1   small onion
1   green pepper
12   black olives, pickled in vinegar
1   purslane, small bunch
1   tbs capers
3   tbs olive oil
1   tbs red wine vinegar
150g   feta cheese
Pinch oregano
Pinch coarse sea salt

Chop tomatoes and cucumbers in a bowl. Cut the onion and the green pepper in rings. Add the olives, capers, oregano, salt and feta. Drizzle with olive oil and vinegar.

Spinach & Mushroom Salad

2 cups spinach
1 cup mushrooms

Chop up spinach. Slice Mushrooms finely and mix together. Toss in dressing of your choice and sprinkle with basil or sunflower seeds.

Cabbage Slaw

1 ½ cups grated cabbage (red or white or both)
1   grated carrot
½   grated green pepper
1 tsp honey
A pinch of celery seeds or crushed black cumin seeds

Toss with salad dressing and serve.

Spicy Pineapple Salad

A few crisp lettuce leaves,
1 fresh pineapple,
2 carrots,
2 sticks celery,
½ green pepper,
2 handfuls of sultanas (or raisins),
½ tsp celery seeds,
1 tsp dry mustard mixed with vinaigrette.

Tear lettuce leaves in a bowl. Peel the pineapple, and cut it into fairly small cubes. Coarsely grate the carrots, and finely chop the celery and green pepper, and add them to the pineapple cubes. Add the sultanas, soaked in water for a few hours to plump them up. Sprinkle with celery seeds. Serve with a piquant mustardy mayonnaise or French dressing.

Orange, Cabbage Salad

4 carrots,
6 oranges,
1-2 cups white cabbage,
2 handfuls of raisins,
4 tsp of sesame seeds.

Coarse chop the carrots. Juice four of the oranges and blend the juice with the carrots until you have a smooth mixture. Finely shred or grate the cabbage and put it in a bowl with the raisins or grapes. Pour the carrot mixture over it and lightly mix with a fork. Sprinkle with the sesame seeds and garnish with the two remaining oranges, peeled and sliced.

Winter's Delight

1 lettuce
6 cherry tomatoes,
1 cup small cauliflower florets,
2 celery stalks finely chopped,
2 carrots (finely grated or cut into matchsticks),
4 radishes sliced,
1 green pepper (cut into thin strips),
Sprigs watercress,
Fresh sweet corn or sprouts to garnish.

Place the lettuce leaves, torn into bite-sized pieces or shredded, into a clear glass bowl. Prepare the vegetables and arrange in layers in the bowl, keeping the watercress for decoration. Dress with a thinned mayonnaise dressing. Top with sweet corn or alfalfa sprouts, and sprigs of watercress.

Avocado & Tomato Salad

1 medium avocado, peeled and chopped
1 medium cucumber, sliced
3 ripe tomatoes,
1 tbs cold pressed olive oil,
1 tbs apple cider vinegar or lemon juice,
Pinch coarse sea salt,
Pinch oregano,

Chop washed and cleaned cucumber and tomatoes in a bowl. Drizzle olive oil and sprinkle with salt and oregano.

Village Salad

4 tomatoes
1 cucumber
1 small onion
1 green pepper
12 black olives, pickled in vinegar
1 purslane, small bunch
1 tbs capers
3 tbs olive oil
150g feta cheese

Pinch oregano
Pinch coarse sea salt
1 tbsp red wine vinegar or apple cider vinegar

Chop tomatoes and cucumbers in a bowl. Cut the onion and the green pepper in rings. Add the olives, capers, oregano, salt and feta. Drizzle with olive oil and vinegar.

Fresh Beetroot & Goat's Cheese Salad.

1kg fresh beetroot (4 bulbs with leaves) (cooked)
Beetroot leaves cooked for 3 minutes
200g green beans (steamed for 3 minutes)
1 tbs red wine vinegar
2 tbs virgin olive oil
1 clove garlic, crushed
1 tbs drained capers, coarsely chopped
100g goat's cheese.

Cut beetroot into thin wedges. Add green beans. Chop beetroot leaves. Crumble goat's cheese over the top and serve.
For the dressing: add red wine vinegar, oil, garlic, capers, ½ tsp each of salt and pepper. Shake pour over salad.

Grated Beetroot with Orange Tarragon Dressing

Ingredients:

¼ cup (50 ml) fresh orange juice
3 tbsp (50 ml) olive oil
1 tsp (5 ml) each of grated orange zest and fresh lemon juice
Liquid Ontario Honey and Dijon mustard
Salt and pepper to taste
3 peeled and finely grated raw Ontario Beets
1 tbsp (15 ml) mixed chopped fresh herbs such as parsley, tarragon, chervil and chives

Fennel & Apple Salad.

2 – 3 red apples, cored and diced
1 medium bulb fennel, tough outer stalk removed, julienned
¼ small red onion, julienned
2 cups arugula or other bitter green, washed and dried

Poppy Seed Dressing:
¼ cup fresh orange juice
1tsp orange zest (preferably organic)
1 tbsp olive oil
1 tsp poppy seeds
¼ tsp herb mare salt

Combine ingredients for the dressing and mix well. Toss all ingredients, except greens. Arrange apple-fennel salad on top of greens and serve.

Sprout and Nut Salad

Romaine lettuce
Lollo rosso (red leafed lettuce)
Spinach leaves
A few sprigs radicchio leaves
½ cup bean sprouts
1 small piece broccoli
2 tbsp fresh ground pumpkin seeds

In a large bowl tear leaves into bite sizes. Steam broccoli until it turns bright green. Hold onto the stem of the broccoli and carefully shave off the flowerets onto the lettuce until only the branches remain. Then take the stems and cut off the hard outer bark on all sides. Slice the stems lengthwise to 1cm and then in half and finely onto 1" lengths. Add sprouts. Toss with dill vinaigrette dressing. Grind pumpkin seeds in coffee / nut grinder and sprinkle over salad.

Garden Salad.

3 handfuls torn romaine lettuce
3 sliced mushrooms
1 handful grated zucchini
4 cucumber slices

1 handful shredded carrot
2 scoops avocado
½ handful sprouts
¼ cup hazelnuts
½ cup raw sunflower seeds and almonds soaked.

Soak sunflower seeds and almonds for at least 3 or more hours. Drain off water and rinse them with fresh water. Arrange the salad together attractively; garnishing with mushroom, sunflower seeds, cashews and almonds. Serve with zesty herb dressing.

Zesty Dressing:
2 1/3 cup olive oil
2/3 cup apple cider vinegar
1 handful basil or parsley finely chopped
2 lemons, juiced
¼ tsp red cayenne
1 tsp thyme
1 stalk celery
1tsp herbed salt
1 bell pepper, finely chopped
1 tbs coarse unprocessed sea salt
Blend in blender. Makes a large jar full. Keeps in refrigerator 2 or 3 days.

Aphrodite's Salad

1 lettuce finely chopped
1 medium avocado, peeled and chopped
1 orange, segments only
1/2 cup raw pistachio nuts

Finely chop lettuce. Add avocado and orange segments. Top with pistachio nuts. This salad is great with mastiha dressing.

Mastiha Dressing

1/3 cup extra virgin Greek olive oil
3   tbsp lemon juice or apple cider vinegar
½ tsp mastiha ground with ½ tsp. salt in a mortar with a pestle
½ tsp oregano
Salt and freshly ground black pepper

Whisk together the olive oil, lemon juice, salt, pepper, oregano and mastiha until a unified emulsion forms.

Greek Chick Pea (Garbanzo) Salad

2 (15 ounce) cans garbanzo beans,
     (or soak overnight and boil your own)
2 cucumbers, halved lengthwise and sliced,
12 cherry tomatoes, halved,
½ red onion, chopped,
2   cloves garlic minced
20 black olives, drained and chopped
1   ounce crumbled feta cheese
½ cup Italian- style salad dressing
½ lemon juiced
½ tsp herbed salt or garlic salt or coarse sea salt
½ tsp ground black pepper

Combine all the ingredients in a large salad bowl. Toss together and refrigerate 2 hours before serving. Serve chilled.

Salad Dressings

Basic Dressings

Please note that one tablespoon of olive oil is 120 calories. For weight management, do not have more than 1 tablespoon of olive oil per meal.

Olive oil, balsamic vinegar,
Olive oil, apple cider vinegar,
Olive oil, lemon juice

To make basic salad dressings more flavourful, you may add salt, pepper, cayenne pepper, paprika, garlic, fresh or dried herbs, mustard or honey.

Tomato Dressing

3-5 tomatoes,
2 tbs lemon juice,
½ tsp basil or parsley

Blend. Store in the fridge for maximum of 3 days.

Avocado & Tomato Dressing

4 small tomatoes,
1 avocado,
2 tbsp lemon juice,
A dash of Tabasco or ½ a hot pepper
1 crushed clove of garlic or a dash of garlic powder.

Mix in a blender. Store in the fridge.

Thousand Island Dressing

1 hard-boiled egg, chopped
5 tsp celery, finely chopped
3 tbsp onion, finely chopped
2 tbsp black olives, chopped
1 tbsp green pepper, finely chopped
½ cup non-fat yoghurt

Mix all the ingredients together and serve chilled.

4 WEEK FOUR

Components of a Healthy Diet

A balanced diet and moderate consumption of foods without regular overeating are likely the most important components of a healthy diet, especially on a long-term basis. Other factors of a healthy diet are:

Natural Foods

The closer our foods are to the garden, fields and orchards the more energy, vitality and nutrients we will obtain. Packaged foods contain chemicals or metals which are toxic. In addition, the packaging is often a costly waste product and may or may not be recycled.

Seasonal Foods

Eating seasonally is important first for providing the right type of fuel to protect us from the climates as our environment provides the best foods to support our health and keep us in balance. For example in summer, the juiciest fruits are available to help cool the body and in the winter we eat richer, heavier foods which helps fuel our bodies to keep us warm and protect us from the cold.

Fresh Foods

Eating fresh foods is one of the healthiest aspects of a diet. This especially applies to fruit, vegetables, grains, nuts, beans and seeds. It also applies to milk and animal products as spoilage or rancidity of the animal foods can easily cause microbial diseases, since bacteria, viruses and parasites grow well in these foods. Most food poisoning cases are caused by protein foods such as eggs, meats, fish, seafood and soft cheeses. The meaning of fresh eating is the short time between a food which has been produced, gathered or prepared for market. The more time which passes the food then becomes less fresh and has to be disposed.

Nutritious Foods

Eating a nutritious diet means acquiring all the vitamins, minerals, amino acids and fatty acids that our body needs to function optimally. It also means eating wholesome foods which contain high levels of nutrients. These once again include, fruit, vegetables, whole grains, legumes, nuts and seeds. The animal foods, though not as balanced can be high in certain important nutrients such as protein, iron, calcium, or vitamin B12.

Clean Foods

Eating a clean diet refers to two important areas. The first part is about consuming chemical-free foods as much as possible. I.e. avoiding chemical additives and chemically treated foods, as well as refined sugar and flour foods. Finding organically grown produce and organic (untreated) poultry, beef, and eggs is becoming more important as pollution worsens in our world.

Clean also refers to washing and storing food properly to avoid spoilage and contamination. Washing fresh produce with *water, salt water solution, white vinegar, mild soap solution or Clorox bleach* aids in removing germs, pesticides, dirt, insects or other chemicals.

Tasty and Attractive Foods

It is important to eat a diet which is tasty, appealing and satisfies our senses. Often to change our diet more positively, we need to work at changing our tastes, or to actually develop new tastes. The unnatural or concentrated sweet or and salty flavours in foods, as well as chemical tastes, have taken people away from simple, natural eating. Adopting a healthy diet may mean that you need to recondition yourself to enjoy the true natural flavours of the real foods of the Earth.

Variety and Rotation

Eating a variety of nutritious foods provides us with a variety of nutrients, thus preventing any obvious deficiencies.

Rotating our diet means eating different foods from day to day and not repeating the same foods every day. This reduces the potential to become allergic or sensitive to particular foods.

Common foods that may cause allergies are: cow's milk, wheat, eggs, soybeans, corn, beef, coffee, chocolate, tomatoes, yeast, shellfish, and mushrooms.

Food Combining

I believe food combining to be an important component to good nutrition. It allows us to digest and utilize the foods and their inherent nutrients optimally. Many people overstress their digestive tracts by eating a large number of foods at each meal, from all the different groups at each sitting. This is very taxing on the body, and may in part be why, in our culture, there is so much digestive disease from stomach to colon. Simple meals of a few ingredients each, using a variety of foods over time, with intent about creating a balanced diet over the day or week is a more healthful overall approach to eating.

The basic principles of food combining are as follows:

1. Starchy foods and sugars (carbohydrates) should not be eaten with proteins or acid fruits at the same meal.
2. Fruit, vegetable and salad foods should form the major part of the diet.
3. Starchy foods and sugars (carbohydrates), proteins and fats should be eaten in small amounts only.
4. Only wholegrain, unrefined carbohydrates should be eaten: all refined, processed foods – in particular white flour, white sugar and their by-products; highly processed fats; sweetened foods; foods containing unnaturally – occurring additives, preservatives and colourings – should be eliminated.
5. There should be an interval of four to four and a half hours between meals of different types.
6. A balance of 80:20 alkali to acid food ratio. Alkali foods are mostly fruits, vegetables, nuts and seeds, yoghurt, milk, – — Acid forming foods – eggs, meat, dairy products, grains,

sugar, honey, vinegar …. It is best to find a table which will show you which are alkali and which are acid forming. They are too many to mention here.

7. Fruits are eaten by themselves or with other fruits and on an empty stomach. I.e. do not eat fruit immediately after a main meal. Melons are best digested when eaten alone and not mixed with other fruits.

8. Proteins and starches are not eaten together. Basic proteins such as meats, poultry, fish, eggs, and milk products require maximum stomach acid levels for best digestion, mainly because of their high fat content. Nuts and seeds also require an acid medium to be digested. Starches or complex carbohydrates are best digested in a relatively more alkaline stomach.

9. Combine protein and vegetables or starch and vegetables.

10. Do not eat more than one protein per meal. Mixing more than one protein, such as eggs and ham can be taxing on the digestive tract and also offers more fat and protein than is needed.

11. Due to its high acidity content. Do not eat cooked tomato dishes more than once a week. Cooked tomato may be eaten with protein dishes rather than carbohydrates.

Moderation

"Pan Metron Ariston" was a common expression in ancient Greece which translates as "all good things in moderation." " Πάν μέτρον άριστον" …

Eating moderately, not overeating or under eating, is probably the basic first habit of nutrition. Eating too much food causes great stress on the body. Regular overeating also tends to reduce our exercise potential, and this, along with the increased calorie intake, contributes to weight increase. Almost all obesity, other than from hormonal imbalance, is caused by overconsumption of calories along with physical under activity. Being overweight, leads to an increase in serious and chronic diseases, such as hypertension, heart disease, diabetes and cancer.

Balance

Eating a balanced diet is probably the most important aspect of nutrition in regard to long-term health. The five aspects of balance are:

- Macronutrients – proteins, fats, and carbohydrates.
- Micronutrients - vitamins, minerals, amino acids, and fatty acids.
- Food Groups – fruits, vegetables, grains, legumes, nuts, seeds, dairy products, eggs, fish, poultry and meats.
- Flavours and Colours
- Acid- alkaline

The Basic Nutrients

Nutrients are substances that are essential for life. The six basic nutrients are carbohydrates, protein, fat, vitamins, minerals, and water. Humans take in these nutrients through food, and if we are deprived of too many nutrients for too long, we weaken, we become ill, and eventually we die.

Water

Water is the basic nutrient, essential for life, whether the life is human, animal, or plant. More than two-thirds of the human body consists of water – and more than two-thirds of the earth's surface is covered by water.

According to Victor Schauberger who has researched water in depth, the best water to drink is fresh spring water coming forth from the earth at cold temperatures (4 degrees Celsius).

Filtered water is best to drink. You may add a squeeze of lemon, lime, green herbs, sea or rock salts or MSM (Methylsulfonylmethane) supplement powder to bring it back to 'life'.

Whenever possible avoid distilled water bottled in plastic. Distilled water is "mineral hungry" and tends to draw substances including plastic into itself. Plastic mimics estrogen (the female sex hormone) inside the body.

Macronutrients and Micronutrients

Of the other five basic nutrients, the carbohydrates, protein, and fat are macronutrients, while vitamins and minerals are micronutrients. The former are called macronutrients because they are essential in large amounts, micronutrients are essential in minute amounts. Both are needed for an organism's proper growth and metabolism.

Macronutrients are the building blocks and energy for the body. *Micronutrients* trigger the mechanisms that replenish the building blocks and ignite the energy.

Carbohydrates are the body's primary source of energy. They fuel the body – its muscle, brain, and central nervous system. The energy in food is measured in calories, and carbohydrates provide four calories per gram. Excess carbohydrate calories are stored in the liver and muscles as glycogen, to be called up when needed as a reserve energy source, or, if not needed, to become fat deposits.

Protein is essential for creating and repairing vital cells and organs. Protein is created in the body from building blocks known as amino acids. There are twenty-two different amino acids that can be assembled in thousands of combinations to provide just the right proteins for an individual's unique needs for organs, muscle, blood, hormones, and enzymes. Fourteen of these amino acids can be manufactured in the body, but the eight-so-called "essential" amino acids must be obtained from food. Protein also provides energy, in the amount of four calories per gram.

Fat is a critical component of cell membranes and hormones and is essential to the process by which some nutrients are absorbed into the system. Fat also cushions organs and helps regulate the body temperature by insulating the body. Fat, too, yields energy: nine calories per gram, more than twice the caloric content of carbohydrates and protein. Powerfoods are an excellent source of essential fatty acids, the building blocks of healthy fat.

Vitamins do much more than prevent disease. They provide the only source of certain co-enzymes necessary for metabolism, the bio-chemical processes that support life. In addition, certain vitamins act as antioxidants – substances that protect the body's cells from the kind of damage that can be caused by pollution, exposure to chemicals, alcohol, and the by-products of normal metabolism. Antioxidants raid the free radicals, the destructive biological molecules that attack cell membranes and cause premature cell death. In their antioxidant role, vitamins are essential in preventing early aging and many of the degenerative diseases.

Minerals are multifunctional within the body, essential to both structure and function. Minerals such as calcium and phosphorus are components of bones and teeth. Magnesium is needed for cellular metabolism, sodium for fluid balance and muscle function, potassium for fluid-electrolyte and acid-base balance, chloride for water balance and digestion, and sulfur for protein structure and enzyme activity.

Humans encounter invasive viruses and can be made weak by stress and pollution. The illnesses that result from these problems take a variety of forms: hypertension, cardiovascular sickness, arthritis, gastrointestinal disorders, cancer and more.
Beyond the body-building, body sustaining power of macronutrients, beyond the sparkplug capabilities of the micronutrients, *phytochemicals* provide essential raw materials for suppressing, retarding, even reversing not just illnesses but also the debilitating effects of stressful contemporary life and the degenerative effects of aging.

Every bite of a *powerfood* is a cocktail containing thousands of these phytochemicals, all of them acting together in mysterious ways to offer a multitude of effects, fighting against the likes of cancer and heart disease while bestowing good health and vitality.

The fact is that humans are genetically programmed to digest and assimilate powerfoods, that is what our natural metabolism was built for. Powerfoods put less stress on the body, requiring less effort for digestion and assimilation even as they put more energy, more good health into the body.

Powerfoods and Phytochemicals Explained

Phytochemicals ("phyto" means plant) are biologically active compounds in plants. To date, scientists have identified over 12,000 phytochemicals. One plant can contain literally hundreds of different types of these compounds.

Of course, the nutritional value of plant foods has long been known, scientific studies as well as common-sense observation confirm that people whose diets are rich in fruits and vegetables live healthier lives.

What scientists are still finding is that a single fruit, vegetable, spice or herb contains thousands of phytochemicals in trace amounts that interact in complex but complementary ways to prevent certain diseases and boost overall health.

It is amazing to think that every bite of a apple, every leaf of a green leafy vegetable, every mushroom contains a rich chemical stew that can, among other things, block, retard, suppress, or flush away carcinogens, lower serum cholesterol and decrease arterial plaque, enhance the immune system, fight the effects of aging.

The Mediterranean Powerfoods

An authentic Mediterranean type diet is rich in whole grains, fruits, vegetables, legumes, fresh and dried herbs, nuts and seeds, walnut, and olive oil, fish and seafood , moderate amounts of red wine. It reduces meat, meat products and refined cereals, sugars and other processed and refined foods.

These are the top groups of food that will create and sustain health. Combinations of these, which appear in the recipes are easy to prepare and delicious to eat:

- Red, yellow, orange and purple fruits
- Red, yellow, orange and purple vegetables
- Cruciferous and leafy green vegetables
- Mushrooms
- Sea Vegetables
- Garlic, onions and company
- Whole grains
- Beans and other legumes
- Nuts and Seeds
- Olives
- Goat's and Sheep's products (yoghurt, sour milk called Airani and cheeses e.g. halloumi, feta, anari)
- Raw unpasteurized honey, bee pollen, royal jelly
- Herbs / Spices
- Seafood and Fish
- Wild Edible Plants
- Sprouts

The Top Sixteen Power Food Groups

Powerfood Group # 1: Red, yellow, orange and purple fruits

Nutrients:　　　　　　　Carotenoids, terpenes, flavonoids, coumarins, vitamin C, boron, fiber

Benefits:　　　　　　　Antioxidants protect vision, prevent degenerative disease (such as arthritis, heart disease, diabetes)

Powerfood Group # 2: Red, yellow, orange and purple vegetables

Nutrients:　　　　　　　Carotenoids, flavonoids, capsaicin, vitamin C, vitamin E, fiber

Benefits: Antioxidants protect vision, prevent degenerative disease (such as arthritis, heart disease, diabetes)

Powerfood Group # 3: Cruciferous and leafy green vegetables

Nutrients: Indoles, carotenoids, isothiocyanates, vitamin C, vitamin E, magnesium, calcium, iron, fiber

Benefits: Neutralize free radicals, stimulate anticancer enzymes, useful in asthma, knock harmful hormones off track.

Powerfood Group # 4: Mushrooms

Nutrients: Lentinan, B Vitamins, copper, fiber

Benefits: Strengthen immune system, antiviral, antitumor, prevent abnormal clotting

Powerfood Group # 5: Sea Vegetables

Nutrients: Carotenoids, vitamin C, calcium, iodine, fiber

Benefits: Promote strong bones, boost metabolism, minimize heavy metal toxicity

Powerfood Group # 6: Garlic and Company

Nutrients: Organosulfur compounds, allicin, quercetin, selenium, phosphorus, iron, potassium, fiber

Benefits: Lower LDL cholesterol, fight infections, fight cancer, boost heart health, anti-inflammatory

Powerfood Group # 7: Whole Grains

Nutrients: Lignans, phenolic acids, phytosterols, B vitamins, vitamin E, magnesium, chromium, fiber

Benefits: Lower cholesterol, help prevent colon cancer, aid in elimination, improve insulin sensitivity, energy source

Powerfood Group # 8: Beans and legumes

Nutrients: Lignans, phenolic acids, phytosterols, B vitamins, vitamin E, magnesium, chromium, fiber

Benefits: Lower cholesterol, help prevent colon cancer, aid in elimination, improve insulin sensitivity, energy source

Powerfood Group # 9: Nuts and Seeds

Nutrients: Lignans, B vitamins, vitamin E, copper, selenium, calcium, essential fatty acids, fiber

Benefits: Boost immune system, lower cholesterol, aid elimination, anti-inflammatory, stimulate enzymes that detoxify

Powerfood Group # 10: Olives

Nutrients: Hydroxytyrosol and oleuropein

Benefits: Inhibits hyperglycemia and oxidative stress induced by diabetes.

Powerfood Group # 11: Goat's and sheep's milk products

Nutrients: Vitamins A, B, and E, calcium, phosphorus, potassium, and magnesium. Short- and medium-chain fatty acids. Conjugated linoleic acid (CLA)

Benefits: Higher proportion of short – and medium –chain fatty acids. They have little effect on cholesterol levels. They also make milk easier to digest. Conjugated linolenic acid (CLA) is a cancer-fighting fat-reducing fat. The fat globules in sheep and goat's milk are smaller than fat globules in cow's milk, making it easier to digest

Powerfood Group # 12: Bee's Products - Honey, Propolis, Pollen and Royal Jelly

Nutrients: Vitamin B1, B2, B3, B5, B6, B12, C, H, inositol, folic acid, amino acids, phosphorous, sulphur. In trace amounts, iron, manganese, nickel, cobalt, silicon, chromium, gold and bismuth

Benefits: Strengthens immune system.

Powerfood Group # 13: Herbs and Spices

Nutrients: Spices and herbs maximize nutrient
                                density. Antioxidants, minerals
                                and multivitamins.

Benefits: Medicinal and culinary uses.

Powerfood Group # 14: Seafood and Fish

Nutrients: B-complex vitamins, calcium,
                                potassium, iodine, zinc, copper,
                                phosphorous and selenium,
                                choline, omega 3 fatty acids, amino
                                acids

Benefits: Brain food, lowers heart disease,
                                cholesterol, controls blood
                                pressure, strengthens immune
                                system

Powerfood Group # 15:   Wild Edible Plants

Nutrients: Wild edible plants maximize
                                nutrients density. Antioxidants,
                                minerals and multivitamins

Benefits: Medicinal and culinary uses

Powerfood Group # 16:   Carob

Nutrients: Phosphorous, calcium,
                                magnesium, potassium,
                                vitamin B2, Vitamin A,
                                folate, choline, selenium

Benefits: Analgesic, anti -allergic, anti-bacterial,
                                antioxidant, antiviral, antiseptic,
                                laxative, lowers cholesterol, combats
                                osteoporosis, prevents lung cancer.

Phytochemicals and Their Benefits

Phytochemicals: Carotenoids (over 600) especially beta carotene, lycopene.

Food Source: Red, green, yellow, orange fruits and vegetables especially carrots, sweet potatoes, winter squash, tomatoes, citrus, melons, cruciferous vegetables.

Benefits: Antioxidants; reduce accumulation of plaque in arteries, promote cell differentiation (cancer cells are undifferentiated).

Phytochemicals: Flavonoids (over 800) especially rutin, hesperidin, and quercetin.

Food Source: Most fruits and vegetables, especially citrus, onions, apples, grapes, tea.

Benefits: Antioxidants that block carcinogens, suppress malignant changes, keep collagen healthy. Protect eyes, nerves from inflammation and damage from diabetes: improve symptoms of allergy, asthma, and arthritis.

Phytochemicals: Ellagic acid

Food Source: Strawberries, grapes, raspberries, apples.

Benefits: Neutralise cancer causing chemicals found in tobacco smoke, processed foods, and barbecued meats.

Phytochemicals: Phenolic Acids

Food Source: Citrus, whole grains, berries, tomatoes, peppers, parsley, carrots, cruciferous vegetables, squash, yams, most other fruits and vegetables.

Benefits: Help resist cancer by inhibiting cell proliferation induced by carcinogens in target organs, inhibit platelet activity, decrease inflammation, and act as antioxidants.

Phytochemicals: Indoles

Food Source: Cruciferous vegetables, such as broccoli, cabbage, kale

Benefits: Block cancer-causing substances before they can damage cells.

Phytochemicals: Isothyocyanates, such as sulforaphane

Food Source: Cruciferous Vegetables

Benefits: Induce protective enzymes; suppress tumor growth

Phytochemicals: Lignans

Food Source: Flax seeds, berries, whole grains

Benefits: Antioxidants and insoluble fibers, block or suppress cancerous changes; anti-inflammatory, particularly protective against colon cancer and heart disease.

Phytochemicals: Saponins

Food Source: Garlic, onions, legumes, soybeans, maca

Benefits: Inhibit tumor promoters induced by excessively fatty diet: lower circulating levels of fats.

Phytochemicals: Protease Inhibitors

Food Source: All plants, especially soybeans

Benefits: Reduce inflammation of arthritis; antiviral and antibacterial; suppress enzyme production in cancer cells, which may slow tumor growth.

Phytochemicals: Terpenes

Food Source: Oranges, lemons, grapefruits

Benefits: Induce protective enzymes, interfere with the action of carcinogens; prevent dental decay; antiulcer activity.

Phytochemicals: Capsaicin

Food Sources: Hot peppers

Benefits: Reduce pain sensation; anti-inflammatory; prevents the activation of cancer-causing chemicals.

Phytochemicals: Coumarins

Food Sources: Soybeans, whole grains, citrus, cruciferous vegetables, cucumbers, squash, melons, parsley, flax seeds, green tea.

Benefits: Anticancer activists; blood thinners.

Phytochemicals: Isoflavones, such as genistein, daidzein

Food Sources: Soybeans, tofu, soy milk

Benefits: Antioxidants that block carcinogens, suppress tumor formation, block estrogen from entering cells to reduce risk of breast and ovarian cancer

Phytochemicals: Organosulfurs, such as allicin, diallyl disulfide

Food Sources: Garlic, onions, leeks, chives, shallots, scallions

Benefits: Block or suppress cancer-causing agents; inhibit cholesterol synthesis, boost immunity, prevent infection. Help resist cancer by inhibiting nitrosamine formation and interfering with cancer-causing enzymes.

Phytochemicals: Phytosterols

Food Sources: Whole grains, legumes, soy

Benefits: Compete with natural estrogens that may promote cancer.

Fiber Foods

Fiber is essential for lowering cholesterol, and research shows that it plays a role in preventing colon cancer. Although fiber is non-nutritive for humans, it is the preferred food of the friendly bacteria that live in our gastrointestinal tracts. Those bacteria in turn produce the short-chain fatty acids that nourish the cells lining our large intestine or colon. The importance of fiber means that it should be a regular part of every diet.

Important Fiber Foods

Grains: Barley, Brown rice, Cracked wheat bread, Oatmeal bread, Oatmeal or rolled oats, White popcorn (plain), popped, Shredded wheat.

Fruits: Apples, Apricots, Cantaloupe, Figs, Grapefruit, Grapes, Oranges, Peaches, Prunes, Raisins, Raspberries.

Nuts and Seeds: Almonds, Pumpkin seeds, Sesame seeds, Sunflower seeds, Walnuts.

Legumes: Dried beans (great northern, kidney, Lima, navy, haricot, black eyed beans), dried peas, Lentils.

Vegetables: Broccoli, Brussels sprouts, Cabbage, Carrots, Cauliflower, Mushrooms, Onions, Potatoes, Sea vegetables (dulse, nori, wakame), Spinach, Squash

Losing Weight with Raw Foods

Losing weight is quite easy when you follow a diet high in raw foods. It is so easy that anyone who has a habit of going on and off slimming diets and achieving only temporary 'success' will be glad to know that on a 75% minimum raw food diet most people lose weight steadily without ever counting calories.

Dr. John Douglass, an experimenter with raw foods in the last fifteen years has voiced that **"For many years I struggled with obesity and was frustrated in treating patients because nothing ever**

seemed to work – not biofeedback or hypnosis or diets or anything. Then I discovered the potential of uncooked foods and found that the more uncooked foods patients used, the less they wanted to eat. These foods are more satisfying for patients and they lose weight on them."

Common weight loss diets are disreputably known to be nutritionally poor. Starting and stopping diets as many dieters do, creates sub-clinical deficiencies that lead to illness and fatigue and also to the 'hidden hunger' that triggers bingeing, bad eating habits and more weight gain.

Raw eating is different. Shedding weight on a raw diet seems to curb the craving for food which causes people to gain weight.
It also improves nutritional status so it encourages steady and continuous loss of those excess pounds.

Being Fat Can Be Harmful !

It is now a scientific fact that being fat predisposes you to serious illnesses such as atherosclerosis, heart disease, high blood pressure, diabetes and cancer, among many others.

Another scientific fact to take into account is that the fatter you get the less efficiently your immune system protects you against infection and early aging.

The question asked is why do so many people overeat when they eat cooked foods, especially junk foods ?
The answer is because their diet is short of vitamins, minerals and other essential nutrients. The body, in a desperate bid for nutritional satisfaction, demands more and more calories.

Overeating produces more toxic wastes than the body can get rid of and so it stows them away in the layer of fat under the skin where they can do as little harm as possible.

The Overburdened Digestive System

An overweight body is a misshaped body with an inherited tendency to store fat. It is nutritionally starved despite the number of calories it has consumed over the years.

Its endocrine system, circulation, bones and nerves are under constant stress.

Overeating too many nutritionally 'void', depleted foods and not eating enough nutritionally rich ones. This leads to the overweight person's digestive system to become overworked. The digestive juices are in overproduction. This leads to deficiencies in important enzymes needed to break down foods fully, provide nutrients needed to break down foods completely and provide nutrients for cell use.

The cells of the body are constantly craving to be fed, plagued by constant appetite, regardless of how much or how little the overweight person puts into his mouth.

The constant stimulation of the digestive organs can result in excess acidity of the stomach and longstanding inflammation of the intestines which further increases the craving for more food.

An overstressed enzymic system can lead to food allergies and result in sub-clinical vitamin and mineral deficiencies which in turn reinforce the vicious circle of hidden hunger. Medicine calls it dysphagia.

Diets Don't Work

Fat cells are much less active than other cells in our body. They burn less energy than muscle cells. This means that the more fat you have relative to muscle the lower your metabolic rate is.
A fat person uses up fewer calories per kilo of body weight than a normal weight person, which is why he or she can eat very little and still not lose weight.

Reducing your calorie intake has much less effect if you are fat.

The Set-Point Theory

- In 1982 Bennet and Gurin originally developed the set-point theory to explain why repeated dieting is unsuccessful in producing long-term change in body weight or shape. Going on a weight-loss diet is an attempt to overpower the set point, and the set point is a seemingly tireless opponent to the dieter.

- The ideal approach to weight control would be a safe method that lowers or raises the set point rather than simply resisting it. So far no one knows for sure how to change the set point, but some theories exist. Of these, regular exercise is the most promising: a sustained increase in physical activity seems to lower the setting (Wilmore et al. 1999).

- According to the set-point theory, the set point itself keeps weight fairly constant, presumably because it has more accurate information about the body's fat stores than the conscious mind can obtain. At the same time, this system pressures the conscious mind to change behavior, producing feelings of hunger or satiety. Studies show that a person's weight at the set point is optimal for efficient activity and a stable, optimistic mood. When the set point is driven too low, depression and lethargy may set in as a way of slowing the person down and reducing the number of calories expended.

- The set point, it would appear, is very good at supervising fat storage, but it cannot tell the difference between dieting and starvation. The dieter who begins a diet with a high set point experiences constant hunger, presumably as part of her body's attempt to restore the status quo. Even dedicated dieters often find that they cannot lose as much weight as they would like. After an initial, relatively quick loss, dieters often become stuck at a plateau and then lose weight at a much slower rate, although they remain as hungry as ever.

- Dieting research demonstrates that the body has more than one way to defend its fat stores. Long-term caloric deprivation, in a way that is not clear, acts as a signal for the body to turn down its metabolic rate. Calories are burned more slowly, so that even a meager diet almost suffices to maintain weight. The body reacts to stringent dieting as thought famine has set in. Within a day or two after semi-starvation begins, the metabolic machinery shifts to a cautious regimen designed to conserve the calories it already has on board. Because of this innate biological response, dieting becomes progressively less effective, and (as generations of dieters have observed) a plateau is reached at which further weight loss seems all but impossible.

(The Center for Health Promotion & Wellness at MIT Medical – Adapted from Integrative Group Treatment for Bulimia Nervosa by Helen Riess, M.D. and Mary Dockray-Miller)

This is not a fixed level but the usual level of fat your body is accustomed to. Whatever weight your body has maintained for, say, a year or so seems to determine your fatpoint. Your body maintains this usual level of fat by checking up hormonally on its fat reserves. The hormones that do this work via the brain, and the level of these hormones in the bloodstream is directly proportional to the amount of fat stored.

It is this fatpoint, and the cravings that are a sign of malnutrition, which spur the familiar phenomenon of rebound eating, uncontrolled eating as soon as you stop dieting.

Rebound eating may raise your fatpoint higher than it was before you began dieting because you have alerted your hormones to the fact that your body's reserves of fat are falling. And so you put on even more weight.

This is how most people's weight creeps up over the years. When you diet repeatedly you are fighting one of your body's most efficient self-protection mechanisms, and you are the one who loses.

The solution is to work with, not against that protection mechanism. You gradually have to readjust your fatpoint so that lost weight stays off.

This means doing three things.

- Eliminating cravings by giving your body all the nutrients it needs (at least 50 essential nutrients are known but fresh raw foods probably contain many more)

- Calming an irritated and overactive digestive system so that its functions return to normal. Then you will derive full benefit from the food you eat and eliminate the ravenous hunger.

- Getting rid of accumulated toxins and amyloid deposits, because these block proper assimilation and adversely affect the endocrine and nervous system.

A diet of well chosen raw foods will do all these things and will do them gradually, without your having to pay attention to calories and without alerting your body's fatpoint defenses.

One of the amazing benefits about losing weight eating large amounts of raw foods is that you do not need to end up looking drawn or flabby.

Skin and muscles becomes firm and the whole body undergoes a slow process of rejuvenation which is little short of miraculous. Most dieters become quite irritable. Flare ups of temper and rapid changes of mood are often due to an over-acid system.

If you have a great deal of fat in your blood, which is usually the case if you are dieting and getting rid of stored fat, your blood will be acidic. Unfortunately most of the foods that make up weight loss diets also increase acidity.

The more acidic your system the more irritable you feel. Raw fresh fruit and vegetables have a counteractive alkalinising effect. This means that you feel calmer, more resilient and less tired while you are losing weight.

Acid/Alkaline Blood Levels

However, most scientists and nutritionists seem to collectively agree that acidic blood is one of the main triggers and or facilitators of many diseases and problems, such as premature aging, stroke, gout, a poor immune system, excessive lethargy and cancer.

Besides, it was also found that blood alkalinity can be enhanced by natural food sources that we have known all along to be healthy, such as fruits and vegetables. So it is pretty much conclusive that alkalized blood is a better and healthier blood status.

Acid/alkaline levels can be measured by pH numbers that range from 1 (the most acidic) to 14 (the most alkaline), with 7 being neutral. Human blood is naturally neutral, with slight alkalinity at a pH level of 7.40. However, because many of us embrace fast food and processed foods in our adult life, we lose our blood alkalinity and start heading towards more acidic blood.

It is believed that alkaline blood contains more hydroxyl ions, which allows our red blood cells to carry more oxygen and white blood cells to be stronger in combating unknown microorganisms that attack our body.

On the other end, acidic blood contains more hydrogen ions, which causes our red blood cells to clump, lowering their ability to carry oxygen and making our white blood cells weaker.

Alkalized blood means less acidic blood, which brings us to your next question about gout. Gout is caused by high level of uric acid in our blood.

Simple logic tells us that alkalized blood will prevent high levels of uric acid. The normal range of uric acid is between 3.0-7.0

milligram/deciliters of blood. It is safer to have a lower score than one near the upper limit of what is considered normal, because uric acid deposits tend to build up in our joints, causing pain and immobility.

Health Tip:

- Avoid drinking water from plastic bottles. Investing in a water filter such as a reverse osmosis filter or carbon filter is well worth it for your health and the environment. You may then store your water in glass bottles.

- Minimise use of sugar, particularly sucrose, or 'white sugar'. Try natural sweeteners, such as date sugar, rice or malt syrup, honey, grape syrup, carob syrup or fructose.

- Use coarse sea salt to flavour your food. Avoid excessive use of salt, refined salt and salty foods.

Meal Preparation Tip:

When preparing meals do not heat up the oil until it is smoking hot. Add oil to pot, keep fire on low heat and immediately add in the onion, garlic or vegetables and let them cook slowly. An ideal temperature for cooking foods in the oven is 180 degrees.

Smoking hot oils (olive oil along with other vegetable oils) increases the amounts of cancer causing polycyclic hydrocarbons PAH's.

Tasks for This Week:

1. This week start food combining. Quite simply don't mix your proteins and starches and all fruits should be eaten on an empty stomach. Fats are neutral and may be eaten with both proteins and carbohydrates.

2. Consume at least one Mediterranean power food each day.

3. Red meat should not be eaten more than once a week or twice at most.

4. Do not eat dishes with cooked tomato more than once a week. It is very acidic for the body.

Complete Meal Plan

Monday
First Thing in the Morning
1 glass lemon water, made with room temperature water
and 1/4 - 1/2 lemon, juiced

Breakfast
Barbara's Nutty Breakfast

Mid-Morning Snack
2 thin slices anari (low fat whey cheese),
drizzle with 1 tsp honey or 1 tbsp carob syrup

OR savoury version

2 thin slices anari cheese
1 tomato
1 cucumber
Drizzle 1/2 tsp olive oil and sprinkle with salt, pepper and oregano.

20 Minutes before Lunch
Drink one or two glasses of water or herbal tea.

Lunch
Spinach Risotto (Spanakorizo) with Greek Salad

Afternoon Snack
1 piece of Fruit a handful of walnuts and 1 -2 dried figs

Dinner
Baked Sardines (or other fish) served with steamed vegetables (i.e.
green beans) and green salad

Evening Snack
2 - 3 squares dark chocolate and an herbal tea

Tuesday
First Thing in the Morning
1 glass lemon water, made with room temperature water
and 1/4 - 1/2 lemon, juiced

Breakfast
1 glass Energy Boost Banana Shake

Mid-Morning Snack
1/2 cup sugar-free muesli
1 tbsp of goat's / sheep's yoghurt,
1/2 tsp honey

20 Minutes before Lunch
Drink one or two glasses of water or herbal tea.

Lunch
Garden Salad top with grilled chicken fillet slices
OR 3/4 cup chick peas

Afternoon Snack
Kefir or Airani and a cucumber.

Dinner
Asparagus and mint frittata served with Tunisian carrot salad

Evening Snack
1 slice goat's cheese and ½ glass red wine

Wednesday
First Thing in the Morning
1 glass lemon water, made with room temperature water
and 1/4 - 1/2 lemon, juiced

Breakfast
1 bowl Banana, Coconut Salad

Mid-Morning Snack
1 boiled egg

1 slice barley, rye or whole grain brown bread
1 tsp butter or mayonnaise or olive oil to spread on bread (optional)
1 cucumber, sliced
1 tomato, sliced
3 olives

20 Minutes before Lunch
Drink one or two glasses of water or herbal tea.

Lunch
Vegetarian dolmades served with Greek salad

Afternoon Snack
1 cup of a selection of Chopped up Vegetables of your choice
(carrots, cucumbers, peppers) + 1 tbsp humus (or other dip such as
tahini or guacamole)

Dinner
Grilled cod steaks with mint pesto serve with avocado and tomato
salad

Evening Snack
6-8 walnut halves drizzled with 1 tsp raw, unprocessed honey

Thursday
First Thing in the Morning
1 glass lemon water, made with room temperature water
and 1/4 - 1/2 lemon, juiced

Breakfast
1 large glass Carob's Delight Smoothie

Mid-Morning Snack
Easy Oat Breakfast

20 Minutes before Lunch
Drink one or two glasses of water or herbal tea.

Lunch
Vegetable Couscous

Afternoon Snack
1 piece of Fruit, a handful of raw almonds and 2 dried apricots.

Dinner
Swiss chard and black eyed bean salad (Louvia me laxana)
Dress with 1 tbsp olive oil and lemon juice apple cider vinegar, salt,
pepper.

Evening Snack
2 - 3 squares dark chocolate and an herbal tea

Friday
First Thing in the Morning
1 glass lemon water, made with room temperature water
and 1/4 - 1/2 lemon, juiced

Breakfast
1-2 pieces of fruit of your choice e.g. 1 peach and 1 apple

Mid-Morning Snack
1 bowl Raw Muesli

20 Minutes before Lunch
Drink one or two glasses of water or herbal tea

Lunch
Whole meal pasta with green pesto sauce and toss in some lightly
steamed broccoli florets serve with cabbage slaw (optional)

Afternoon Snack
1 piece of Fruit, a handful of raw pistachios and a handful of sugar-
free cranberries

Dinner
Celery soup served with slice of rye, barley or whole wheat brown
bread

Evening Snack
Two banana oat cookies an herbal tea

Saturday
First Thing in the Morning
1 glass lemon water, made with room temperature water
and 1/4 - 1/2 lemon, juiced

Breakfast
1 glass Oat, Banana and Pear smoothie

Mid-Morning Snack
2 thin slices goat's cheese like feta or halloumi or anari
1 slice barley, rye or whole grain brown bread
1 cucumber, sliced
1 tomato, sliced
1 tsp olive oil or butter
Sprinkle oregano, salt and pepper

20 Minutes before Lunch
Drink one or two glasses of water or herbal tea.

Lunch
Mediterranean fish stew served with brown rice and steamed
broccoli and carrots

Afternoon Snack
1 piece of Fruit, a handful of raw hazelnuts and 2 small dates

Dinner
French oven roasted vegetables served with quinoa or brown rice
and a green salad (optional)

Evening Snack
One slice of halloumi (1cm thick) + ½ glass red wine

Sunday

First Thing in the Morning
1 glass lemon water, made with room temperature water
and 1/4 - 1/2 lemon, juiced

Breakfast
1-2 pieces of fruit of your choice e.g. 1 peach and 1 apple

Mid-Morning Snack
Omelet with 2 -3 eggs and vegetables of your choice like
mushrooms, spinach, asparagus, onions, peppers etc.
1 tbsp grated goat's cheese
Serve with cucumber and tomato slices.
3 olives

20 Minutes before Lunch
Drink one or two glasses of water or herbal tea.

Lunch
Lemon & Coriander Baked lamb served with roast potatoes and a
village salad

Afternoon Snack
A dessert of your choice like a slice of chocolate or carrot cake, 2
scoops ice-cream or a fruity yoghurt.

Dinner
Mushroom Soup

Evening Snack
2 -3 squares dark chocolate and an herbal tea

General Rules And Guidelines.

a) With regards to the main meals. I do realize that most people lead very busy lives and it is next to impossible to prepare two meals a day. What you can do is prepare one main meal for dinner and eat leftovers for lunch the next day. You can also get imaginative and where appropriate you can use some leftovers from dinner as a salad topping for lunch. Get creative !

b) Remember to eyeball your portion of lean meat, poultry, or fish – it should be about the size of your palm and fish 3/4 of your hand.

c) Bread Choices: Choose dark brown whole wheat bread, rye, barley, spelt. No more than one slice per day.

d) Avoid the white processed carbohydrates and very starchy vegetables such as potatoes, white rice and white pasta. If you do eat them no more than a portion the size of a **tennis ball.**

e) Cheese servings are about the size of a matchbox or the size of your thumb.

f) Raw, stir-fried, steamed, baked or grilled vegetables, and are unlimited - you may eat as much as you want.

g) Herbal teas are drunk throughout the day.

h) Fried foods are to be avoided and rarely eaten.

Recipes

Please note that I have added a few extra recipes which you may swop for other meals found on the meal plan.

Mushroom Soup
serves 4

1kg Fresh mushrooms (use whichever ones are in season)
4   spring onions, finely chopped
1   small onion
1   small bunch dill, finely chopped
1   organic egg
¼   cup cold pressed olive oil
2tbs white dry wine
1   lemon juiced
4   cups water
Pinch green pepper

Clean mushrooms very well and make sure that all soil has been removed. Cut the mushrooms into small pieces and set aside to dry. Add the olive oil in a pot and sauté the onions till lightly browned. Then add the mushrooms and keep stirring for 1 – 2 minutes. Add in the white wine, and immediately after add four cups of water. Cover and simmer for 20 minutes.

Add in the spring onions, dill and stir well for an additional 15 minutes. Add in the pepper and the salt to taste. Turn off the heat.

In a glass bowl beat egg until frothy. Keep beating the egg and very slowly add a tablespoon of lemon juice and then a couple of tablespoons of broth from the soup, keep alternating until all the lemon juice has been used.

Add the mixture to the remaining soup and stir well. Soup is served hot, with pepper and a little finely chopped dill.

Swiss chard and Black eyed bean salad
serves 6

600g   black eyed beans
1 kg   chard or beet tops or spinach
¼ cup   olive oil
2   lemons, juiced.

Soak the black eyed beans in water for at least 8 hours. Rinse. Place in a pot with boiling water and simmer for about 30 minutes until cooked. Wash and clean the chard removing and tough stalks. Add to the pot and cook for a further 5 to 6 minutes. When cooked place in a dish. Place in a jar the lemon juice, olive oil and salt. Shake well and pour over the bean salad.

Celery soup – dairy free version
serves 4

1 lb   celery hearts
1   small red onion
1   small potato
4 cups vegetable stock
2 tbs   cold-pressed olive oil
2   bay leafs

Method:

Peel and chop onion and potato. Sautee with olive oil in a 3-quart saucepan until tender. Add vegetable stock and bring to boil. Chop celery and add to saucepan along with bay leafs. Turn the heat down to low and simmer for 30 minutes. Remove bay leafs from soup. With a soup ladle put about half of the mixture in the blender. Hold the lid on securely while pureeing for one minute. Repeat with the other half of the mixture. Stir all the soup together well.

Plain Bean Salad
serves 6

550g dried white beans
1   medium onion
4 tbs cold pressed extra virgin olive oil
2 tbs lemon juice
4 tbs chopped parsley
Salt

Soak beans in water for at least 10 hours. Wash and drain. Boil in water for 30 minutes or until cooked. Drain and place in a bowl. Add salt, onion, olive oil, lemon juice and sprinkle with parsley.

Fennel salad with yoghurt
serves 4

1 cup fresh fennel hearts, chopped
1   cucumber diced
1 cup radishes diced
2 cups strained yoghurt or goat's sheep's yoghurt
1 tsp fresh mint finely chopped
1   lemon juiced
Pinch of salt
Pinch of white pepper freshly ground

Add all the ingredients to a bowl, mix and serve.

Vegetarian Dolmades
makes 24

200g   vine leaves in brine
1 cup medium – grain rice
1   small onion, finely chopped
1 tbs olive oil
60g   pine nuts
2 tbs currants
2 tbs chopped fresh dill
1 tbs finely chopped fresh mint
1 tbs finely chopped fresh flat-leaf parsley
1/3 cup olive oil

2 tbs   lemon juice
2 cups vegetable stock

1. Soak the vine leaves in cold water for 15 minutes, then remove and pat dry. Cut off any stems. Reserve some leaves to line the saucepan and discard any that have holes or look poor. Meanwhile, soak the rice in draining water for 10 minutes to soften, and then drain.
2. Place the rice, onion, 1/3 cup olive oil, pine nuts, currants, herbs and salt and pepper, to taste, in a large bowl and mix well.
3. Lay some leaves vein –side-down on a flat surface. Place 1 tablespoon of filling in the centre of each, fold the stalk end over the filling into the centre, and finally roll firmly towards the tip. The dolmades should resemble a small cigar. Repeat with the remaining filling and leaves.
4. Use the reserved vine leaves to line the base of a large, heavy-based saucepan. Drizzle with 1 tablespoon olive oil. Add the dolmades, packing them tightly in one layer, then pour the remaining oil and lemon juice over them.
5. Pour the stock over the dolmades and cover with an inverted plate to stop the dolmades moving around while cooking. Bring to the boil, then reduce the heat and simmer, covered, for 45 minutes. Remove with a slotted spoon. Serve warm or cold. These can be served with lemon wedges.

Note: Unused vine leaves can be stored in brine in an airtight container in the fridge for up to a week.

French Oven Roasted Vegetables
serves 4

4   new potatoes, cleaned and cut into 1" chunks
12   large mushrooms cut into halves
1   medium eggplant, sliced into 1 1/2 "square chunks
2   zucchini, sliced 1 ½" thick
1   large onion, quartered and separated
2   red bell peppers, seeded and cut into 1 ½"square pieces
4   cloves garlic minced
1 tsp paprika
½ tsp onion powder
Olive oil cooking spray

Celtic sea salt to taste
Freshly ground black pepper

Toss all ingredients except oil, salt, and pepper, making sure to coat each vegetable with seasoning.
Spray baking sheet with olive oil spray and place vegetables evenly on top. Bake for 30 to 40 minutes in a preheated 375 degree oven. Season to taste with salt and pepper and arrange attractively on each plate. Serve hot or room

Mediterranean Fish Stew
serves 4

3 tbsp	olive oil
2	onions, sliced
2	carrots sliced
3	celery sticks, sliced
125g	mushrooms, sliced
2	garlic cloves
4	tomatoes, skinned and chopped
300ml	dry white wine
600ml	fish or vegetable stock
1	bay leaf
750g	cod or haddock fillet, skinned and boned
200g	jar of mussels in brine, drained
175g	peeled prawns

Salt and pepper
Chopped parsley, to garnish

Heat the oil in a large saucepan and add the onions, carrots, celery, mushrooms and garlic. Cook until softened, but not brown. Add the tomatoes, wine, stock and bay leaf. Season with salt and pepper to taste and simmer for 15 minutes.
Cut the fish into 5cm cubes. Add them to the saucepan and simmer for 15 minutes. Add the mussels and prawns and simmer for another 2 – 3 minutes. To serve, turn the stew into a warmed serving dish and garnish with the chopped parsley.

Spanakorizo (Spinach Risotto)
serves 3

Ingredients:

2 1/4	pounds of fresh spinach, chopped, washed, drained
1	spring onion, chopped
2 tbs	olive oil
1 1/3	cup of water
1 1/3	cups of long-grain rice (optional use quick cook brown rice)
5 1/4	cups of water
	sea salt and freshly ground pepper
	juice of 1 lemon (about 2 tablespoons)

Preparation:

In a stock pot, sauté the chopped spring onion in the oil over medium heat for 8-10 minutes. Add spinach and 1 1/3 cups of water and cook until the spinach wilts, about 5-7 minutes. Add rice and 5 1/4 cups of water, bring to a boil, and cook for 15 minutes, stirring occasionally. Stir in lemon juice and salt, cook for another 5 minutes and remove from heat. Stir, cover, and let sit for 20 minutes until the dish "melds." Try topping with a sprinkle of crumbled feta.

Mushroom Risotto
serves 4

20g	dried porcini mushrooms
1 litre	vegetable stock
2 tbs	olive oil
100g	butter, chopped
650g	small cap or Swiss brown mushrooms, stems, trimmed, sliced
3	cloves garlic, crushed
1/3	cup dry white vermouth
1	onion, finely chopped
2	cups risotto rice
1 ½	cups grated parmesan

Soak the porcini mushrooms in 2 cups warm water for 30 minutes. Drain, retaining the liquid. Chop them and pour the liquid through a fine sieve lined with a paper towel. Put the stock and the mushroom liquid together in a saucepan, bring to the boil, then reduce heat, cover and keep at a low simmer. Heat half the oil and 40g of butter. Add the mushrooms and the garlic to the pan and cook, stirring, for 10 minutes, or until soft and all the mushroom juices have been released. Reduce heat to low and cook for another 5 minutes or until all the juices have evaporated. Increase the heat, add the vermouth and cook for 2-3 minutes, until evaporated. Set aside. Heat the remaining olive oil and 20g butter in a large saucepan over medium heat. Add the onion and cook until soft. Add rice and stir for 2 minutes. Add ½ cup stock to the pan and stir constantly until liquid is absorbed. Continue adding more stock ½ cup at a time until tender and creamy. Remove from heat and stir in the mushrooms, Parmesan and the remaining butter. Season, to taste, with salt and freshly ground black pepper.

Spinach with Raisins and Pine Nuts
serves 3

500g   spinach
2 tbs   pine nuts
1 tbs   olive oil
1   small red onion, halved and sliced
1   clove garlic, thinly sliced
2 tbs   raisins
Pinch of ground cinnamon

Trim the stalks from the spinach and discard. Wash the leaves and shred them. Put the pine nuts in a frying pan and stir over medium heat for 3 minutes, or until lightly brown. Remove from the pan. Heat the oil in the pan, add the onion and cook over low heat, stirring occasionally, for 10 minutes, or until translucent. Increase the heat to medium, add the garlic and cook for 1 minute. Add the spinach with the water clinging to it, the raisins and cinnamon. Cover and cook for 2 minutes, or until the spinach wilts. Stir in the pine nuts, and season, to taste.

Note: Silver beet (Swiss chard) works equally well in this recipe, although it may take a little longer to cook than the spinach.

Artichokes with garlic and herb butter
serves 4

2   large or 4 medium globe artichokes
    pinch salt and white pepper

For the garlic and herb butter:

75g butter
1   garlic clove, crushed
1   tbsp mixed chopped fresh tarragon, marjoram and parsley

Steam artichokes until tender. In a pan sauté garlic in butter for 1 or 2 minutes over low heat, add the artichokes, and herbs. Mix well and serve.

Grilled Cod Steaks with mint pesto
serves 4

4 cod steaks about 6 oz each
Olive oil to baste
Lemon juice
Salt and pepper
Lime wedges to garnish

Mint Pesto

6 tbs chopped mint
1 tbs chopped parsley
1   garlic clove
1 tbs grated Parmesan cheese
1 tbs single cream
1 tsp balsamic vinegar
3 tbs extra virgin olive oil

Brush the cod with oil and squeeze over a little lemon juice. Season with salt and pepper and cook under a preheated moderate grill for 3 – 4 minutes on each side until golden and cooked through.

Meanwhile place all the ingredients for the pesto in a blender or food processor and blend until fairly smooth. Season with salt and pepper to taste and transfer to a bowl. Alternatively, pound the ingredients together with a mortar and pestle. Serve the cod steaks topped with a spoonful of the pesto and green beans, if liked. Garnish with lime wedges.

Lentil Moussaka
serves 4

3 tbs	olive oil
1	onion, chopped
4	celery sticks, chopped
1	garlic clove, crushed
400g	can chopped tomatoes
250g	green lentils
2tbs	Japanese Soy Sauce
900ml	water
500g	aubergines, sliced
1 tbs	grated Parmesan Cheese
1 tbs	oregano to garnish

Salt and pepper

Topping:
2 eggs, beaten
150ml low-fat fromage frais

Heat one tablespoon of the oil in a saucepan, add the onion and cook until softened. Add the celery, garlic, tomatoes with their juice, lentils, soy sauce, ¼ teaspoon pepper and water. Cover and simmer for 50 minutes, until cooked.

Heat the remaining oil in a griddle pan, add the aubergine slices in batches and cook on both sides until golden. Alternatively, cook under a preheated moderate grill.

Cover the base of a shallow ovenproof dish with the lentil mixture and arrange a layer of aubergine slices on top. Repeat the layers, finishing with a layer of aubergines slices.

Mix the topping ingredients, season with salt and pepper to taste, and pour over the aubergines. Top with the cheese and bake in a preheated moderate oven at 180 degrees for 30-40 minutes until golden. Serve garnished with oregano.

Baked Zucchini
serves 4

8   small zucchini, about 450g
15ml   olive oil, plus a little extra for greasing
100g   goat's cheese, cut into thin strips (feta may be used)
        small bunch fresh mint, finely chopped
        freshly ground black pepper

Preheat the oven to 180 degrees C. Trim the zucchini and cut a thin slit along the length of each. Insert pieces of goat's cheese (feta) in the slits. Add a little mint and sprinkle with the olive oil and black pepper. Cover and bake for 25minutes until tender.

Shrimp with Tomatoes, Feta and Ouzo
serves 4

1/2   cup extra-virgin olive oil
2   tbs minced garlic
2   (28-ounce) cans Italian plum tomatoes,
        crushed with your hands, with juices
1/2   cup bottled clam juice or seasoned shrimp stock
2 1/2 tsp minced fresh oregano leaves
1 1/2 tsp minced fresh thyme leaves
1 1/4 tsp crushed red pepper flakes
1/4   cup drained small capers
        salt and pepper
5   tablespoons unsalted butter
2   pounds raw large shrimp, peeled and deveined
1/2   cup ouzo
1/2   pound Greek Feta cheese, crumbled

Hot crusty peasant-style bread, for serving

Directions

In a large saucepan heat the olive oil and, when hot, add the garlic and cook until fragrant, about 1 minute. Add the tomatoes, clam juice, oregano, thyme, crushed red pepper, and capers, and cook until the sauce is thickened and reduced by half in volume, 20 to 25 minutes.
Season, to taste, with salt and pepper and set aside.
Preheat the oven to 350 degrees F.

Heat the butter in a large skillet until it begins to foam. Add the shrimp and cook, stirring occasionally, until they just begin to turn pink. Remove pan from heat, and add ouzo. Return pan to the heat and shake carefully to ignite the alcohol. Season lightly with salt, to taste. Remove from the heat. Do not overcook; shrimp should not be cooked through at this point.

Add the sauce to a large casserole dish or individual gratin dishes. Nestle the shrimp down in the sauce and crumble the feta evenly over the top. Bake for 12 to 15 minutes or until shrimp are cooked through and the sauce is hot and bubbly. Remove from the oven and serve immediately, with pieces of crusty bread for dipping.

Stuffed Whole Calamari (Kalamaria Yemista)
serves 4

1kg medium squid with hoods whole
4 large ripe tomatoes or 1 can tomatoes
1 tbsp olive oil
1 onion finely chopped
1 clove garlic
¼ cup red wine
1 tbsp fresh chopped oregano

Stuffing:
1 tbsp olive oil
2 spring onions, chopped
1 ½ cups cold cooked rice
60 g pine nuts
75g currants
2 tbsp chopped fresh parsley
2 tsp finely grated lemon rind
1 egg lightly beaten

Preheat the oven to warm 160 degrees. For the tomato sauce, chop tomato flesh or can of peeled tomatoes. Heat the oil in a frying pan over medium to low heat. Add the onion and garlic and cook over low heat for about 2 minutes, stirring frequently, until the onion is soft. Add the tomato, wine and oregano and bring to the boil. Reduce the heat, then cover and cook over low heat for 10 minutes.

Meanwhile, for the stuffing, mix all the ingredients except the egg in a bowl. Add enough egg to moisten the ingredients.

Wash the squid and pat dry with paper towels. Three –quarters fill each hood with the stuffing and secure the ends with toothpicks or skewers. Place in a single layer in a casserole dish.

Pour the tomato sauce over the squid, cover the dish and bake for 20 minutes, or until the squid are tender. Cut the squid into thick slices. Spoon the sauce over just before serving.

NOTE: You will need to cook ½ cup rice for this recipe. The cooking time for the squid will depend upon the size. Choose small squid because they are more tender.

Asparagus and mint frittata
serves 4

6	eggs
1/3 cup	grated Pecorino or Parmesan
¼ cup	fresh mint leaves, finely shredded
200g	baby asparagus spears
2 tbs	extra virgin olive oil

Put the eggs in a large bowl, beat well, then stir in the cheese and mint and set aside.

Trim the woody part off the asparagus then cut the asparagus on the diagonal into 5cm (2 inch) pieces. Heat the oil in a 20cm (8inch) frying pan that has a heatproof handle. Add the asparagus and cook for 4-5 minutes, until tender and bright green. Season with salt and pepper, and then reduce the heat to low.

Pour the egg mixture over the asparagus and cook for 8 – 10 minutes. During cooking, use a spatula to gently pull the sides of the frittata away from the sides of the pan and tip the pan slightly so the egg runs underneath the frittata.

When the mixture is nearly set but still slightly runny on top, place the pan under a low grill for 1 – 2 minutes, until the top is set and just browned. Serve warm or at room temperature.

Serve salad or steamed vegetables.

Note: There are very many variations of frittatas. You can make them with
zucchini, red pepper, green beans, broccoli, spinach or any leftover
vegetables you have from the previous day.

Chicken Cacciatore
serves 4

¼	cup olive oil
1	large onion, finely chopped
3	cloves garlic, crushed
150g	pancetta finely chopped
125g	button mushrooms
1	large chicken cut into 8 pieces
1/3 cup	dry vermouth or dry white wine
2 x 400g	cans chopped tomatoes
¼ tsp	soft brown sugar
¼ tsp	cayenne pepper

1 sprig of fresh oregano
1 sprig of fresh thyme
1 bay leaf

Heat half the olive oil in a large heatproof casserole dish. Add the onion
and garlic and cook for 6 – 8 minutes over low heat, stirring, until the
onion is golden. Add the pancetta and mushrooms, increase the heat and
cook, stirring for 4 – 5 minutes. Transfer to a bowl.

Add the remaining oil to the casserole dish and brown the chicken pieces, a
few at a time, over medium heat. Season with salt and black pepper as they
brown. Spoon off the excess fat and return all the chicken to the casserole
dish. Increase the heat, add the vermouth to the dish and cook until the
liquid has almost evaporated.

Add the chopped tomato, brown sugar, cayenne pepper, oregano, thyme
and bay leaf, and stir in 1/3 cup water to the dish. Bring to the boil, then
stir in the reserved onion mixture. Reduce the heat, cover and simmer for
25 minutes, or until the chicken is tender but not falling off the bone.

If the liquid is too thin, remove the chicken from the casserole dish,
increase the heat and boil until the liquid has thickened. Discard the sprigs

of herbs and adjust the seasoning. Can be garnished with fresh oregano or thyme sprigs and served with steamed rice.

Baked Sardines
serves 2

Preheat the oven to 180 degrees.

Place about six cleaned sardines in an oven proof dish, large enough to fit them snuggly in one layer.

Season with salt and ½ tsp pepper. Drizzle with 3 tablespoons oil and 2 tablespoons lemon juice and sprinkle with 1 small chopped clove garlic and 1 ½ teaspoons dried oregano.

Turn to coat, then bake, uncovered, in the top half of the oven for about 15 – 20 minutes, or until the flesh flakes and starts to come away from the bones. Serve hot or warm with lemon wedges.

Octopus Stifado

1kg octopus
1/3 cup olive oil
1kg onions, chopped
1/3 cup vinegar
2 -3 cloves garlic
3-4 bay leaves
Pinch of pepper

Wash the octopus and chop into small pieces. Sauté onions in olive oil for 2 – 3 minutes, then add the octopus. Cook over low heat for 20 minutes. Add in the garlic, vinegar, bay leaves, pepper and a little water if needed and cook till tender.

Tunisian Carrot Salad
serves 6

500g carrots, thinly sliced
3 tbs finely chopped fresh flat-leaf parsley
1 tsp ground cumin
1/3 cup olive oil

¼ cup	red wine vinegar
2 cloves	garlic, crushed
¼ to ½	tsp harissa (mixture of spices can be bought from delicatessens)
12	black olives
2	hard-boiled eggs, quartered

Bring 3 cups water to the boil in a saucepan. Add the carrot and cook until tender. Drain and transfer to a bowl. Add the parsley, cumin, olive oil, vinegar and garlic. Season with harissa, salt and pepper. Stir well.

To serve, place the carrots in a serving dish and garnish with the olives and eggs.

Note: If the carrots are not sweet, you can add a little honey to the dressing. Also, if you prefer a non-spicy version, omit the harissa.

Vegetable Couscous
serves 4 – 6

3 tbs	olive oil
2	small onions, thinly sliced
1 tsp	turmeric
½ tsp	chili powder
2 tsp	grated fresh ginger
1	cinnamon stick
2	carrots, thinly sliced
2	parsnips, thickly sliced
1 ½	cups vegetable stock
315g	pumpkin, cut into small cubes
250g	cauliflower, cut into small florets
2	zucchini, cut into thick slices
425g	can chickpeas, drained
2 tbs	fresh chopped coriander
2 tbs	fresh chopped parsley
1 ¼	cups instant couscous
1	cup boiling water
30g	butter
Pinch of saffron threads	

Heat 2 tbsp of the oil in a large saucepan. Add the onion and cook over medium heat for 5 minutes, or until the onion is soft, stirring occasionally.

Add the turmeric, chili powder and ginger and cook, stirring, for another minute.

Add the cinnamon stick, carrot, parsnip and stock to the pan and stir to combine. Cover and bring to the boil. Reduce the heat and simmer for 5 minutes, or until the vegetables are almost tender.

Add the pumpkin, cauliflower and zucchini and simmer for another 10 minutes. Stir in the chickpeas, saffron, coriander and parsley and simmer, uncovered, for 5 minutes. Remove the cinnamon stick.

Place the couscous in a bowl and add the boiling water. Cover, allow to stand for 5 minutes, and then add the remaining oil and butter and fluff with a fork. Place a bed of couscous on each serving plate and top with the vegetables.

Note: Almost any seasonal vegetables can be used in this recipe. Potato, orange sweet potato, green beans, baby onions, or red or green peppers (capsicums) are all suitable.

Lemon and Coriander Baked Lamb

1.8kg	leg of lamb
2	cloves garlic, sliced
3	large strips lemon rind, cut into 1 cm pieces
½	cup chopped fresh coriander
3 tbs	chopped fresh parsley
2 tbs	olive oil

Preheat the oven to moderate 180 degrees. Trim the lamb of excess fat and sinew. Using a sharp knife, make deep cuts in the flesh and place a slice of garlic and a piece of lemon rind into each cut.

Combine the coriander, parsley, oil and 1 tsp ground black pepper. Coat the lamb with the herb mixture and place on a rack in a baking dish. Pour 1 cup water into the dish and bake for 1 hour 20minutes or until the lamb is cooked to your liking. Add extra water to the pan while cooking if the lamb starts to dry out. Serve the lamb in slices with pan juices and vegetables in season.

Banana-Nut Oatmeal Cookies

2   cups rolled oats
1/2   cup chopped walnuts, pecans, or sunflower seeds
1   cup raisins
3   medium bananas
2½   tbs butter, melted
2 ½   tbs flaxseed or walnut oil
1/4   cup orange juice

Preheat the oven to 180C. Line an oven tray with grease proof paper. In a large bowl, combine the rolled oats, nuts, and raisins. Put the bananas, melted butter, oil and orange juice in a blender. Blend until you have a smooth liquid. Add the liquid mixture to the oat mixture and mix well, until the oats have absorbed the liquid and are fairly soft. Drop the dough by the tablespoonfuls onto the tray. Leave 1/2 inch between them, Bake for 20 - 25 minutes, or until brown around the edges. Cool on a rack.

5 WEEK FIVE

Herbs and Spices

The World Health Organization estimates that 80 per cent of the earth's population today depends on plants to treat common ailments. The medicinal use of herbs is said to be as old as mankind itself. In early civilizations, food and medicine were linked and many plants were eaten for their health-giving properties. Herbs are free from toxicity and addiction. They are organic substances and not manmade synthetic molecules, they possess an affinity for the human organism. They are extremely efficient in balancing the nervous system, restoring a sense of wellbeing and relaxation which is necessary for optimum health and for the process of self-healing.

Using Common Medicinal Mediterranean Herbs

A few common herbs and spices which are not native to the Mediterranean have been included for their medicinal and culinary purposes.

Commercial herbs are available in many different forms. You may buy them in bulk, herb blends, teas, oils, tinctures, fluid extracts, tablets and capsules.

A practical and easy way of incorporating herbs in your daily routine is by drinking them as teas, making infusions and using their essential oils.

Teas, Infusions and Decoctions

People have been consuming herbal teas for as long as they have known how to heat water. Herbal teas can be made from virtually any plant, and from any part of the plant, including the roots, flowers, seeds, berries or bark, although there are some herbs, such as Echinacea, gingko leaf, saw palmetto and milk thistle that have no effective effect when taken in tea form because their active components are not water soluble, and the concentration needed for medicinal potency is so high it can be obtained only from an extract pill, or capsule.

Herbal teas are very good at relieving mild to moderate ailments such as upset stomach, sore throat, coughs, stuffy nose and insomnia.

Many herbals teas are available in tea bag form. They can also be prepared from the fresh herb. To make an herbal tea, place the leaves, flowers roots or bark into a small pot. Pour boiling water over them and allow them to steep for four to six minutes. Some herbs may need a full twenty minutes to steep in order to deliver their full therapeutic effect.

A simple way of preparing teas is to place the herb or herbs in a large 1 ½ liter thermos, pour boiling water over them, close the thermos and let them steep for a minimum of twenty minutes. Drink the tea throughout the day. You may even top up the thermos a second time or third time. It's a wonderful way of keeping hydrated throughout the day.

Infusion is simply another term for tea. This is the easiest way to take herbal remedies. To make an infusion you simply boil water and add leaves, stems, flowers, or powdered herbs – plant material whose active ingredients dissolve readily in hot water – then steep, strain, and drink the mixture as a tea.

A decoction is a tea made from thicker plant parts, such as bark, roots, seeds, or berries. These also contain lignin, a substance that is difficult to dissolve in water. Thus, decoctions require a more vigorous extraction method than infusions.

Essential oils are highly concentrated extracts typically obtained either by steam distillation or cold pressing from the flowers, leaves, roots, berries, stems, seeds, gums, needles, bark, or resins of numerous plants. They contain natural hormones, vitamins, antibiotics, and antiseptics.

It is best to use essential oils externally only, such as in poultices, inhalants, bath water, or on the skin (two to three drops diluted in one tablespoon of a base oil such as almond oil).

The therapeutic properties of essential oils can help to remedy ailments ranging from insomnia to respiratory disorders to impotence to arthritis.

Most herbs act gently and subtly. They do not produce the kind of dramatic, immediate results we expect from prescription drugs. Basically, herbs are balancers that work with the body to help it heal and regulate itself. They work better together than they do singly because the effect of one herb is usually supported and reinforced when combined with others.

While most herbs aren't likely to be harmful, keep in mind that "natural" isn't a synonym for "safe".

Like synthetic drugs, herbal preparations may be toxic, cause allergic reactions, or affect your response to other medications. Common sense, care, and forethought are needed when using herbs for either food or medicine.

Here are some essential guidelines for herbal self-care:

- Use herbal self-care for minor ailments only, not for serious or life-threatening conditions.

- Use only recommended amounts for recommended periods of time.

- Use the correct herb. Buy your herbal remedies from a reputable company. If you collect or grow herbs on your own, be absolutely positive in your identification.

- Use the correct part of the plant. For instance, don't substitute roots for leaves. When buying fresh herbs, check to be sure which part of the herb is required for a remedy – the whole herb, flowers, fruit, leaves, stems, or roots.

- When using an herbal remedy for the first time, start with a small amount to test for possible allergic reactions.

- Don't take certain herbs if you are pregnant or planning to become pregnant

- Don't take herbal remedies if you are nursing a baby.

- Don't give medicinal amounts of herbs to children without first consulting with your health care practitioner.

Herbs and Their Uses

The following table describes some of the most commonly used medicinal herbs, including which parts of each herb are used, its chemical and nutrient content, and it's various uses.

Herb (Scientific Name)	Nutrient Content	Action and Uses	Comments
Alfalfa (Medicago sativa) **Parts Used:** Flowers, leaves, petals, sprouted seeds	Calcium, copper, folate, iron, magnesium, manganese, phosphorous, potassium, silicon, zinc, vitamins A, B1, B2, B3, B5, B6, C, D, E, and K.	Alkalises and detoxifies the body. Acts as a diuretic, anti-inflammatory, and antifungal. Lowers cholesterol, balances blood sugar and hormones, and promotes pituitary gland function. Good for anemia, arthritis, ulcers, bleeding-related disorders, and disorders of the bones and joints, digestive system, and skin.	Must be used in fresh raw form to provide all nutrients. Sprouts are especially effective (be sure to rinse them thoroughly before use to remove mold and bacteria).
Aloe (Aloe Vera) **Parts Used:** Pulp from insides of succulent leaves.	Amino acids, calcium, folate, iron, magnesium, phosphorous, potassium, zinc, vitamins A, B1, B2, B3, C, and E.	Acts as an astringent, emollient, antifungal, antibacterial, and antiviral. Applied topically, heals burns and wounds, and stimulates cell regeneration. Ingested, helps to lower cholesterol, reduces inflammation resulting from radiation therapy, increases blood-vessel generation in lower extremities of people with poor circulation, soothes stomach irritation, aids	Allergic reactions, though rare, may occur in susceptible persons. Before using, apply a small amount behind the ear or on the underarm. If stinging or rash occurs, do not use. Warning: Should not be taken internally during pregnancy.

		healing, and acts as a laxative. Good for AIDS and for skin and digestive disorders.	
Anise (Pimpinella anisum) **Parts Used:** Seeds, seed oil.	Calcium, iron, magnesium, manganese, phosphorous, potassium, zinc, vitamins A, B1, B2, B3, B5, B6, C, and E.	Aids digestion, clears mucus from air passages, combats infection, and promotes milk production in nursing mothers. Good for indigestion and for respiratory infections such as sinusitis. Also helpful for menopausal symptoms.	Used in many popular products as a fragrance and flavouring.
Basil (Ocimum Basilicum) **Parts Used:** Leaves, oil	Good source of protein, Vitamin E (Alpha Tocopherol), Riboflavin and Niacin, and a very good source of Dietary Fiber, Vitamin A, Vitamin C, Vitamin K, Vitamin B6, Folate, Calcium, Iron, Magnesium, Phosphorus, Potassium, Zinc, Copper and Manganese.	Reduces stress, enhances stamina, relieves inflammation, lowers cholesterol, eliminates toxins, protects against radiation, prevents gastric ulcers, lowers fevers, improves digestion and provides a rich supply of antioxidants and other nutrients. Basil is especially effective in supporting the heart, blood vessels, liver and lungs and also regulates blood pressure and blood sugar.	
Bay Leaf (*Laurus nobilis*) **Parts Used:** Leaves, oil	Copper, potassium, calcium, manganese, iron, selenium, zinc and magnesium. Vitamin C, vitamin A, folic acid and niacin, pyridoxine, pantothenic acid and riboflavin.	It has astringent, diuretic, and appetite stimulant properties. Soothe the stomach and relieve flatulence and colic pain. The lauric acid in the bay laurel leaves has insect repellent properties. Bay laurel infusions are used to soothe the stomach ulcers and relieve flatulence. The components in the essential oil can also be used in many traditional medicines in the treatment of arthritis, muscle pain, bronchitis and flu symptoms.	Warning: Should not be used during pregnancy as it may cause miscarriage.
Black Walnut (Juglans nigra)	Calcium, iron, magnesium, manganese,	Aids digestion and acts as a laxative. Helps heal mouth and throat sores. Cleanses	When boiled, the hulls, produce a dye that is used to color

Parts Used:	phosphorous, potassium, selenium, silicon, zinc, vitamins B1, B2, B3, and C.	the body of some types of parasites. Good for bruising, fungal infection, herpes, poison ivy, and warts. May help lower blood pressure and cholesterol levels.	wool.
Husks, inner bark, leaves, nuts.			
Burdock (Arctium lappa) **Parts Used:** Plant, roots, seeds.	Amino Acids, calcium, copper, chromium, iron, magnesium, manganese, phosphorous, potassium, selenium, silicon, zinc, vitamins B1, B2, B3, and C.	Acts as an antioxidant. May help to protect against cancer by helping control cell mutation. Aids elimination of excess fluid, uric acid, and toxins. Has antibacterial and antifungal properties. Purifies the blood, restores liver and gallbladder function, and stimulates the digestive and immune systems. Helps skin disorders such as boils and carbuncles, and relieves gout, and menopausal symptoms. Burdock root used as a hair rinse promotes scalp and hair health.	Warning: Interferes with iron absorption when taken internally.
Calendula (Calendula officinalis) **Parts Used:** Flower Petals	Calcium, coenzyme Q10, vitamins C and E.	Reduces inflammation and is soothing to the skin. Helps regulate the menstrual cycle and lower fever. Useful for skin disorders, such as rashes and sunburn, as well as for neuritis and toothache. Good for diaper rash and other skin problems in small children.	Also called pot marigold. Usually nonirritating when used externally.
Cayenne (Capsicum frutescens or C. annum) **Parts Used:** Berries	Amino acids, calcium, essential fatty acids, folate, iron, magnesium, phosphorous, potassium, zinc, vitamins B1, B2, B3, B5, B6, C, and E.	Aids digestion, improves circulation, and stops bleeding from ulcers. Acts as a catalyst for other herbs. Good for the heart, kidneys, lungs, pancreas, spleen, and stomach. Useful for arthritis and rheumatism. Helps to ward off colds, sinus infections, and sore throats. Good for pain when applied topically. Used with lobelia for nerves.	Also called capsicum, hot pepper, red pepper. Note: Avoid contact with the eyes.
Celery (Apium Graveolens) **Parts Used:** Plant, roots, seeds.	Amino acids, boron, calcium, choline, essential fatty acids, folate, inositol, iron, magnesium, manganese, phosphorous, potassium,	Reduces blood pressure, relieves muscle spasms, and improves appetite. Good for arthritis, gout, and kidney problems. Acts as a diuretic, antioxidant, and sedative.	Warning: The seeds should not be used during pregnancy, nor should large amounts of the herb.

	selenium, sulfur, zinc, vitamins A, B1, B2, B3, B5, B6, C, E and K.		
Chamomile (Matricaria recutita or M. chamomilla)

Parts Used:

Flowers, plant. | Choline, vitamins B1, B3, and C. | Reduces inflammation, stimulates the appetite, and aids digestion and sleep. Acts as a diuretic and nerve tonic. Helpful for colitis, diverticulosis, fever, headaches, and pain. Good for menstrual cramps. A traditional remedy for stress and anxiety, indigestion, and insomnia. Useful as a mouthwash for minor mouth and gum infections. | Also called German chamomile, wild chamomile. Roman chamomile. Caution: should not be used daily for long periods of time, as this may lead to ragweed allergy. Should be used with caution by those who are allergic to ragweed. Should not be used with sedatives or alcohol. |
| Cinnamon (Cinnamomum verum)

Parts Used:

Bark, Plant. | Calcium, chromium, copper, iodine, iron, manganese, phosphorous, potassium, zinc, vitamins A, B1, B2, B3, and C. | Relieves diarrhea and nausea, counteracts congestion, aids peripheral circulation. Warms the body and enhances digestion, especially the metabolism of fats. Also fights fungal infection. Useful for diabetes, weight loss, yeast infection, and uterine hemorrhaging. | Warning: Should not be used in large amounts during pregnancy. |
| Clove (Syzygium aromaticum)

Parts Used:

Flower buds, essential oil. | Calcium, iron, magnesium, manganese, phosphorous, potassium, zinc, vitamins A, B1, B2, and C. | Has antiseptic and anti-parasitic properties. Acts as a digestive aid. Essential oil is applied topically for relief of toothache and mouth pain. | Warning: Clove oil is very potent and can cause irritation, if used in its pure form. Dilute oil in a base oil like olive oil is advised. Essential oil should NOT be taken internally. |
| Dandelion (Taraxacum officinale)

Parts Used:

Flowers, leaves, roots, tops | Calcium, iron, magnesium, manganese, phosphorous, potassium, selenium, zinc, vitamins B1, B2, B3, and C. | Acts as a diuretic. Cleanses the blood, liver and increases bile production. Reduces serum cholesterol, uric acid levels. Improves functioning of the kidneys, pancreas, spleen, and stomach. Relieves menopausal symptoms. Useful for abscesses, anemia, boils, breast tumours, cirrhosis of the liver, constipation, fluid retention, hepatitis, jaundice, and rheumatism. Believed to help prevent age spots and | Leaves can be boiled and eaten like spinach (young leaves can be used in salads). Warning: Should not be combined with prescription diuretics. Not recommended for people with gallstones or biliary tract obstruction. |

		breast cancer.	
Elder (Sambucus nigra) **Parts Used:** Flowers, fruit, inner bark, leaves, roots	Calcium, essential fatty acids, vitamins A, B1, B2, B3, and C.	Combats free radicals and inflammation. Relieves coughs and congestion. Builds the blood, cleanses the system, and eases constipation. Enhances immune system function, increases perspiration, lowers fever, soothes the respiratory tract, and stimulates circulation. Effective against flu viruses. Flowers may be used to soothe skin irritations.	Warning: Should NOT be used during pregnancy. The stems of this plant should be avoided. They contain cyanide and can be very toxic.
Fennel (Foeniculum vulgare) **Parts Used:** Fruit, roots, stems	Amino acids, calcium, choline, essential fatty acids, iron, magnesium, manganese, phosphorous, potassium, selenium, vitamins B1, B2, B3, C, and E.	Used as an appetite suppressant and as an eyewash. Promotes the functioning of the kidneys, liver, and spleen, and also clears the lungs. Relieves, abdominal pain, colon disorders, gas, and gastrointestinal tract spasms. Useful for acid stomach. Good after chemotherapy and / or radiation treatments for cancer.	The powdered plant can be used as a flea repellent.
Fenugreek (Trigonella foenum-graecum) **Parts Used:** Seeds	Amino acids, calcium, essential fatty acids, folate, iron, magnesium, manganese, phosphorous, potassium, selenium, zinc, vitamins B1, B2, B3 and C.	Acts as a laxative, lubricates the intestines, and reduces fever. Helps lower cholesterol and blood sugar levels. Helps asthma and sinus problems by reducing mucus. Promotes lactation in nursing mothers. Good for the eyes and for inflammation and lung disorders.	
Feverfew (Chrysanthemum parthenium) **Parts Used:** Bark, dried flowers, leaves	Calcium, iron, magnesium, manganese, phosphorous, potassium, selenium, zinc, vitamins B1, B2, B3, and C.	Combats inflammation and muscle spasms. Increases fluidity of lung and bronchial tube mucus, promotes menses, stimulates the appetite, and stimulates uterine contractions. Relieves nausea and vomiting. Good for arthritis, colitis, fever, headaches, migraine headaches, menstrual problems, muscle tension, and pain.	Warning: Should not be used during pregnancy. People who take prescription blood-thinning medications or who regularly take over-the-counter painkillers should consult a health care provider before using feverfew, as the combination can result in internal

			bleeding.
Flax (Linum usitatissimum) **Parts Used:** Seeds, seed oil	Amino acids, calcium, essential fatty acids, iron, magnesium, manganese, phosphorous, potassium, sulfur, vanadium, zinc, vitamins B1, B2, B3, B5, and E.	Promotes strong bones, nails, and teeth, as well as healthy skin. Useful for colon problems, female disorders, and inflammation.	The seeds are an excellent addition to a diet that is low in fiber.
Garlic (Allium sativa) **Parts Used:** Bulb	Calcium, folate, iron, magnesium, manganese, phosphorous, potassium, selenium, zinc, vitamins B1, B2, B3, and C.	Detoxifies the body and protects against infection by enhancing immune function. Lowers blood pressure and improves circulation. Lowers blood lipid levels. Helps stabilize blood sugar levels. Aids in the treatment of arteriosclerosis, arthritis, asthma, cancer, circulatory problems, colds and flu, digestive problems, heart disorders, insomnia, liver disease, sinusitis, ulcers, and yeast infections. May prevent ulcers by inhibiting growth of Helicobacter pylori, the ulcer-causing bacterium. Good for virtually any disease or infection.	Garlic contains many sulfur compounds, which give it its healing properties. Odorless garlic supplements are available. Warning: NOT recommended for people who take anticoagulants, as garlic has blood thinning actions.
Gentian (Gentiana lutea) **Parts Used:** Leaves, roots	Calcium, iron, magnesium, manganese, phosphorous, potassium, selenium, zinc, vitamins B1, B2, B3, and C.	Aids digestion, stimulates appetite, and boosts circulation. Kills worms and plasmodia (organisms which cause malaria). Good for circulatory problems and pancreatitis.	
Ginger (Zingiber officinale) **Parts Used:** Rhizomes, roots	Amino acids, calcium, essential fatty acids, iron, magnesium, manganese, phosphorous, potassium, selenium, zinc, vitamins, B1, B2, B3, B6, and C. Ground ginger also contains vitamin A.	Fights inflammation, cleanses the colon, reduces spasms and cramps, and stimulates circulation. A strong antioxidant and effective antimicrobial agent for sores and wounds. Protects the liver and stomach. Useful for bowel disorders, circulatory problems, arthritis, fever, headache, hot flashes, indigestion, morning sickness, motion sickness, muscle pain, nausea, and vomiting.	Can cause stomach distress if taken in large quantities. Warning: Do not take if you use anticoagulants or have gallstones. Not recommended for extended use during pregnancy.

Goldenseal (Hydrastis Canadensis) **Parts Used:** Rhizomes, roots	Calcium, iron, magnesium, manganese, phosphorous, potassium, selenium, zinc, vitamins B1, B2, B3, and C.	Fights infection and inflammation. Cleanses the body. Increases the effectiveness of insulin and strengthens the immune system, colon, liver, pancreas, spleen, and lymphatic and respiratory systems. Improves digestion, regulates menses, decreases uterine bleeding, and stimulates the central nervous system. Good for allergies, ulcers, and disorders affecting the bladder, prostate, stomach, or vagina. Used at the first sign of possible symptoms, can stop a cold, flu, or sore throat from developing.	Warning: Do not use if pregnant or breastfeeding. Should not use for prolonged periods of time.
Green Tea (Camellia sinensis) **Parts Used:** Leaves	Amino acids, calcium, iron, magnesium, manganese, phosphorous, potassium, zinc, vitamins B1, B2, B3, B5, and C.	Acts as an antioxidant and helps to protect against cancer. Lowers cholesterol levels, reduces the clotting tendency of the blood, stimulates the immune system, fights tooth decay, helps regulate blood sugar and insulin levels, combats mental fatigue, and may delay the onset of artherosclerosis. Good for asthma. Shows promise as a weight-loss aid. May help prevent enlarged prostate.	Drink without milk. The milk may bind with the beneficial compounds making them unavailable to the body. Warning: Contains caffeine. Should not be used by pregnant or breastfeeding women. Also persons suffering from anxiety disorder or irregular heartbeat should drink no more than 2 cups per day.
Hawthorn (Crataegus laevigata) **Parts Used:** Flowers, fruit, leaves	Amino acids, calcium, choline, chromium, essential fatty acids, iron, magnesium, manganese, phosphorous, potassium, selenium, silicon, zinc, vitamins B1, B2, B3, and C.	Dilates the coronary blood vessels, lowers blood pressure and cholesterol levels, and restores heart muscle. Decreases fat deposit levels. Increases intracellular vitamin C levels. Useful for anemia, cardiovascular and circulatory disorders, high cholesterol, and lowered immunity.	
Hops (Humulus lupulus) **Parts Used:**	Amino acids, calcium, chromium, magnesium, potassium,	Relieves anxiety. Stimulates the appetite. Useful for cardiovascular disorders, hyperactivity, insomnia, nervousness, pain,	Placed inside a pillowcase, aids sleep. Warning: Do NOT use if taking

Flowers, fruit, leaves.	selenium, silicon, zinc, vitamins B1, B3, and C.	restlessness, sexually transmitted diseases, shock, stress, toothaches, and ulcers.	antidepressants.
Horehound (Marrubium vulgare) **Parts Used:** Flowers, leaves	B-complex vitamins, iron, potassium, vitamins A, C, and E.	Decreases thickness and increases fluidity of mucus in the bronchial tubes and lungs. Boosts the immune system. Useful for indigestion, loss of appetite, bloating, and hay fever, sinusitis, and other respiratory disorders.	Warning: Large doses may cause irregular heart rhythms.
Horsetail (Equisetum arvense) **Parts Used:** Stems	Nutrients: Calcium, iron, magnesium, manganese, phosphorous, potassium, selenium, silicon, zinc, vitamins B1, B2, B3, and C.	Acts as a diuretic, lessens inflammation, and reduces muscle cramps and spasms. Aids calcium absorption, which promotes healthy skin and strengthens bone, hair, nails and teeth. Bolsters healing of broken bones and connective tissue. Strengthens the heart and lungs. Useful for the treatment of arthritis, bone diseases, such as osteoporosis and rickets, bronchitis, cardiovascular disease, edema, gallbladder disorders, gout, muscle cramps, and prostate disorders. Used in poultice form to depress bleeding and accelerate healing of burns and wounds.	Also called bottle brush, shave grass. If this herb is used for a long period, supplemental vitamin of B1 (thiamin), should be taken, as horsetail interferes with the absorption of this vitamin.
Lavender (Lavandula angustifolia) **Parts Used:** Flowers		Relieves stress and depression. Beneficial for the skin. Good for burns, headaches, psoriasis, and other skin problems.	
Lemon Balm / Melissa ((*Melissa Officinalis*)		Antispasmodic – eases menstrual pains and tension as well as other emotional issues related to the menstrual cycle, antiviral, antibacterial, mild diaphoretic, carminative, nervine, tonic. Melissa is most affective for nervous system disorders also. The herb is also good for the digestive system (reduces	

		flatulence, indigestion and colic). It is a mild sedative yet it uplifts the mood making it an ideal herb for depression.	
Mastiha (Pistacia lentiscus Mastic)	Nutrients: Triterpenoids	Indigestion, including stomach pain, upper abdominal pain and heartburn. Stomach and intestinal ulcers. Kills H. Pylori. Gum disease, Crohn's disease, Breathing problems, Muscle aches, Bacterial and fungal infections, Repelling insects, hypertension, Cuts, when applied to the skin.	
Milk Thistle (Silybum marianum) **Parts Used:** Fruit, leaves, seeds.	Nutrients: calcium, fatty acids, iron, magnesium, manganese, phosphorous, potassium, selenium, zinc.	Protects the liver from toxins and pollutants by preventing free radical damage and stimulates the production of new liver cells. Also protects the kidneys. Good for gallbladder and adrenal disorders, inflammatory bowel disorders, psoriasis, weakened immune system, and all liver disorders. Has shown anticancer effects against prostate cancer and breast cancer.	Also called Mary Thistle, wild artichoke. Because milk thistle has poor water solubility, it is not effective as a tea. A concentrated capsule or extract form is best.
Mullein (verbascum Thapsus) **Parts Used:** Leaves	Nutrients: calcium, iron, magnesium, manganese, phosphorous, potassium, selenium, zinc, vitamins B1, B2, B3, and C.	Acts as a laxative, painkiller, and sleep aid. Taken internally, aids in getting rid of warts. Clears congestion. Useful for asthma, bronchitis, difficulty breathing, earache, hay fever, and swollen glands. Used in kidney formulas to soothe inflammation.	
Mustard (Brassica nigra) **Parts Used:** Seeds		Improves digestion and aids in the metabolism of fat. Applied externally, helpful for chest congestion, inflammation, injuries and joint pain.	Warning: Can be irritating when applied directly to the skin. Not recommended for use on children under the age of six.
Nettle (Urtica dioica)	Nutrients: Calcium, copper,	Acts as a diuretic, expectorant, pain reliever,	Also called stinging nettle.

Parts Used: Flowers, leaves, roots	fatty acids, folate, iron, magnesium, manganese, phosphorous, potassium, selenium, sulfur, zinc, vitamins B1, B2, B3, B5, C, and E.	and tonic. Good for benign prostatic hyperplasia, anemia, arthritis, rheumatism, hay fever, and other allergic disorders, kidney problems, and malabsorption syndrome. Improves goiter, inflammatory conditions, and mucous conditions of the lungs. Used in hair care products, helps stimulate hair follicles and regulate scalp oil buildup.	
Oat Straw (Avena sativa) **Parts Used:** Whole plant	Nutrients: calcium, folate, iron, magnesium, manganese, phosphorous, potassium, selenium, zinc, vitamins A, B1, B2, B3, B5, B6 and E.	Acts as an antidepressant and restorative nerve tonic. Increases perspiration. Helps to ease insomnia. Good for bed-wetting, depression, stress, and skin disorders.	
Parsley (Petroselinum crispum) **Parts Used:** Fruit, leaves, roots, stems	Calcium, folate, iron, magnesium, manganese, phosphorous, potassium, selenium, zinc, vitamins A, B1, B2, B3, B5, C, and E.	Contains a substance that prevents the multiplication of tumour cells. Expels worms, relieves gas, stimulates normal activity of the digestive system, and freshens breath. Helps bladder, kidney, liver, lung, stomach, and thyroid function. Good for bed-wetting, fluid retention, gas, halitosis, high blood pressure, indigestion, kidney disease, obesity and prostate disorders.	Contains more vitamin C than oranges by weight.
Peppermint (Mentha piperita) **Parts Used:** Flowering tops, oil, leaves	Calcium, choline, iron, magnesium, manganese, phosphorous, potassium, selenium, zinc, vitamins B1, B2, B3, and E.	Increases stomach acidity, aiding digestion. Slightly anesthetizes mucous membranes and the gastrointestinal tract. Useful for chills, colic, diarrhea, headache, heart trouble, indigestion, irritable bowel syndrome, nausea, poor appetite, rheumatism, and spasms.	Warning: May interfere with iron absorption. Should not be used by nursing mothers. Do not ingest pure menthol or pure peppermint leaves.
Primrose (Oenothera biennis) **Parts Used:**	Amino acids, calcium, essential fatty acids, iron, magnesium, manganese,	Promotes cardiovascular health. Aids in weight loss and reduces high blood pressure. Acts as a natural estrogen promoter. Helpful in	Also called evening primrose. Warning: Primrose root should NOT be used during pregnancy.

Seed oil	phosphorous, potassium, vitamin E, zinc.	treating alcoholism, arthritis, hot flashes, menstrual problems such as cramps and heavy bleeding, multiple sclerosis, and skin disorders.	
Pumpkin (Cucurbita pepo) **Parts Used:** Flesh, seed	Amino acids, calcium, essential fatty acids, iron, magnesium, manganese, phosphorous, potassium, selenium, zinc, vitamins A, c, and E.	Useful for prostate disorders and irritable bladder.	
Rose (Rose canina) **Parts Used:** Fruit(hips)	Calcium, iron, magnesium, manganese, phosphorous, potassium, selenium, zinc, vitamins B1, B2, B3, C, and E.	Good for bladder problems and all infections. A good source of vitamin C when used fresh. Rose hip tea is good for diarrhea.	Many vitamin and other supplements are derived from rose hips.
Rosemary (Rosmarinus officinalis) **Parts Used:** Leaves	Calcium, iron, magnesium, manganese, phosphorous, potassium, zinc, vitamins B1, B3, and C.	Fights free radicals, inflammation, bacteria and fungi. Relaxes the stomach, stimulates circulation and digestion, and acts as an astringent and decongestant. Improves circulation to the brain. Also helps detoxify the liver, and has anticancer and antitumour properties. Good for headaches, high and low blood pressure, circulatory problems, and menstrual cramps. Can be used as an antiseptic gargle.	Makes a good food preservative. Warning: Should not be used during pregnancy.
Sage (Salvia officinalis) **Parts Used:** Leaves	Boron, calcium, iron, magnesium, manganese, phosphorous, potassium, selenium, zinc, vitamins B1, B2, B3, B5, and C.	Stimulates the central nervous system and digestive tract, and has estrogenic effects on the body. Reduces sweating and salivation. Good for hot flashes and other symptoms of estrogen deficiency, whether in menopause or following a hysterectomy. Beneficial for disorders affecting the mouth and throat, such as tonsillitis. In tea form, can be used as a hair rinse to promote shine (especially dark hair) and hair growth. Also used to dry up	Warning: Interferes with the absorption of iron and other minerals when taken internally, and when decreases milk supply in nursing mothers. Should not be taken by individuals with seizure disorders. Should not be taken during pregnancy.

		milk when women wish to stop nursing.	
St. John's Wort (Hypericum perforatum) **Parts Used:** Flowers, leaves, stems, oil.	Vitamin C	Good for depression and nerve pain. Helps control stress. In laboratory studies, protects bone marrow and intestinal mucosa from x-ray damage. Applied topically, the oil aids wound healing.	Warning: Large amounts can cause heightened sun sensitivity, especially in light-sensitive people. Should not be used by people who take prescription anti-depressants or any medication that interacts with MAO inhibitors... Should be used with caution during pregnancy.
Thyme (Thymus vulgaris) **Parts Used:** Berries, flowers, leaves	Amino acids, calcium, essential fatty acids, iron, magnesium, manganese, phosphorous, potassium, selenium, zinc, vitamins B1, B2, B3, and C.	Eliminates gas and reduces fever, headache, and mucus. Has strong antiseptic properties. Lowers cholesterol levels. Good for asthma, bronchitis, croup and other respiratory problems, and for fever, headache, and liver disease. Eliminates scalp itching and flaking caused by candidiasis.	
Valerian (Valeriana officinalis) **Parts Used:** Rhizomes, roots	Calcium, choline, essential fatty acids, iron, magnesium, manganese, phosphorous, potassium, selenium, zinc, vitamins B1, B2, B3, and C.	Acts as a sedative, improves circulation, and reduces mucus from colds. Good for anxiety, fatigue, high blood pressure, insomnia, irritable bowel syndrome, menstrual and muscle cramps, nervousness, pain, spasms, stress, and ulcers.	A water-soluble extract form is best. Warning: Should not be combined with alcohol.
Vervain (Verbena officinalis) **Parts Used:** Flowers, leaves, shoots, stems		Strengthens the nervous system. Promotes liver and gallbladder health. Reduces tension and stress. Induces sweating. Promotes menstruation and increases mother's milk. Useful for mild, depression, insomnia, headache, toothache, wounds, colds, fever.	Warning: Do NOT use during pregnancy as it stimulates uterine contractions.
Wild Oregano (Origanum vulgare) **Parts Used:**	Calcium, essential fatty acids, iron, magnesium, manganese, phosphorous,	Fights free radicals, inflammation, and bacterial, viral, and fungal infection. Boosts the immune system. Useful for acne, allergies,	Oregano sold in supermarkets is usually a combination of several oregano

	potassium, zinc, vitamins A, B1, B3, and C.	animal bites, arthritis, asthma, athlete's foot, bee stings, bronchitis, chronic infections, cold, cough, diarrhea, digestive problems, earache, eczema, fatigue, gum disease, headache, menstrual irregularities, muscle pain, parasitic infections, psoriasis, sinusitis, skin infections, urinary tract disorders, and wounds.	species, and does not have the medicinal benefits of Origanum vulgare.
Leaves, shoots, stems			
Wormwood (Artemisia absinthium) **Parts Used:** Leaves, tops.	Vitamin C	Acts as a mild sedative, eliminates worms, increases stomach acidity, and lowers fever. Useful for loss of appetite and liver, gallbladder, gastric, and vascular disorders, including migraine. Applied topically, good for healing wounds, skin ulcers and blemishes, and insect bites.	Often used with black walnut for the removal of parasites. Warning: Should not be used during pregnancy as it can cause spontaneous abortion. Can be habit-forming with long-tem use.
Yellow dock (Rumex crispus) **Parts Used:** Roots	Calcium, iron, magnesium, manganese, phosphorous, potassium, selenium, zinc, vitamins B1, B2, B3, and C.	Acts as a blood purifier and cleanser, and as a general tonic. Improves colon and liver function. Good for inflammation of the nasal passages and respiratory tract, anemia, liver disease, and skin disorders, such as eczema, hives, psoriasis, and rashes. Combined with sarsapilla, makes a tea for chronic skin disorders.	Also called curled dock. Warning: Yellow dock leaves should not be consumed in soups or salads. They are high in oxalates and may cause oxalic acid poisoning.

Yucca (Yucca baccata) **Parts Used:** Roots	Calcium, iron, magnesium, manganese, phosphorous, potassium, selenium, zinc, vitamins B1, B2, B3, and C.	Purifies the blood. Beneficial in treating arthritis, osteoporosis, and inflammatory disorders.	Routinely prescribed for arthritis in some clinic. Can be cut up, added to water (1 cup of yucca in 2 cups of water), and used as a soap or shampoo substitute. Can be added to shampoo also.

Quick Guide to Using Herbs.

As you will often see one herb is helpful for several conditions:

For indigestion / stomach ache – peppermint, caraway, dill, fennel, aniseed, lemon balm

Diuretics for weight loss / for the kidneys – celery seed, marsh mallow, dandelion, golden rod, agrimony

For the liver – dandelion, rosemary

For infections / colds – rose hip, comfrey, aniseed, sage

Diaphoretic for producing a sweat and reducing a fever – lime / linden, peppermint, elderflower, yarrow

Sleep inducing / calming the nerves – lavender, chamomile, hops, lime, orange blossom, passion flower, valerian

As a tonic – nettle, mint, ginseng, rosemary, blackberry, raspberry and strawberry leaf

Skin Disorders – golden rod, St. John's Wort

Health Tip:

Delicious mixtures of herb teas can be found in health food shops.
You may find them sold packaged as tea bags or in loose form.
It is best to buy organic herbs grown without pesticides and
herbicides.

Tasks for This Week:

1. Add in at least three cups of herbal tea a day. You may
   consider purchasing a large thermos to prepare large batches
   of tea which may last you throughout the day.

6 WEEK SIX

The Nutrition Delusion

We are surrounded by a vast array of foods claiming to be healthy. Is it possible that this overwhelming variety of foods is not providing us with everything we need ?

In today's world, a typical diet of supermarket food falls well short of optimum nutrition. Yet paradoxically our need for nutrition is much higher in order to deal with the added pollution we face every day.

Not surprisingly our health is suffering. We are suffering from over 160 nutrient deficiency diseases. The conditions killing us now in huge numbers are not viruses and bacteria, but preventable degenerative conditions such as heart disease, cancer, Alzheimer's, Parkinson's disease and diabetes.

We all begin with a basic genetic blueprint. This gives us weak spots or predispositions to various conditions, such as heart disease, diabetes, asthma etc. But genetics accounts for maybe 20% of illness. The rest of the 80% illness is determined by environmental factors.

Our health is the result of the interaction of our inherited strengths, weaknesses and our circumstances.

Nutrients are the essence of life. Many sources say we need over 90 nutrients every day to function well. These include 60 minerals, 16 vitamins, 12 amino acids and 3 essential fatty acids. We obtain these from the foods we eat.

There are two main factors affecting the level of nutrients in our bodies. They are:

- What we put into our bodies in the form of food or nutrition
- The toxic level of the environment we live in making demands on our nutrients.

Wholefood Supplements — Your Health Insurance

Whole, organic, minimally processed foods are always the preferred choice. There can be no substitute for healthy eating. Yet given our polluted and stress filled world it can be difficult, if not impossible to get our full quota of nutrients in our diet. We can still look to nature for supplements that are plant derived and from natural sources.

Finding a source of good quality supplements is essential.
It is best to avoid synthetic nutrients as they are isolated compounds such as vitamins and minerals produced in a laboratory. Natural supplements may contain other beneficial nutrients not yet discovered; luckily our bodies know what they are for.
Artificial additives and fillers can also be a problem. Supplements that are not labeled natural may also include coal tars, artificial colouring, preservatives, sugars and starch.

This means that like any consumer item, quality can come at a price. Cheap products have lower nutrient levels and more harmful fillers and additives. Good quality supplements may give you expensive urine, but they also give you expensive blood.

Investing in your health brings quality of life !

Nature Knows Best

In nature each food is a whole food, meaning that it has a perfect combination of vitamins, minerals, enzymes, essential fatty acids plus many unidentified phytonutrients. But, as mentioned earlier, this is a far cry from what ends up on our plate. Many foods have most of the nutrients refined out to improve shelf life. Some of the macro minerals are the only ones replaced. This then can leave us getting virtually none of the many microminerals such as boron, selenium, manganese, or sulphur. As the name suggests, microminerals are ones we need only small amounts of and their deficiencies affect us gradually or in more subtle ways.

Listed Below Are Some Whole Food Supplements with their Actions and Uses

Name:	Aloe Vera
Nutrient Content:	Amino acids, calcium, folate, iron, magnesium, phosphorous, potassium, zinc, vitamins A, B1, B2, B3, C, and E.
Action and Uses:	Aid in the healing of stomach disorders, ulcers, constipation, hemorrhoids, rectal itching, colitis, and all colon problems. Helpful against infections, varicose veins, skin cancer, and arthritis and AIDS.
Comments:	Allergic reactions, though rare, may occur in susceptible persons. Before using, apply a small amount behind the ear or on the underarm. If stinging or rash occurs, do not use. **Warning:** Should not be taken internally during pregnancy.
Name:	Barley Grass
Nutrient Content:	Calcium, iron, all essential amino acids, chlorophyll, flavonoids, vitamin B12, vitamin C, plus many minerals and enzymes.

Action and Uses:	Heals stomach, duodenal and colon disorders as well as pancreatitis. Anti-inflammatory.

Name: Bee Pollen

Nutrient Content: B complex vitamins, vitamin C, essential fatty acids, enzymes, carotene, calcium, copper, iron, magnesium, potassium, manganese, sodium, plant sterols, and simple sugars.

Action and Uses: Heals stomach, duodenal and colon disorders as well as pancreatitis. Anti-inflammatory.

Comments: Antimicrobial, combats fatigue, depression, cancer, colon disorders. Helpful for people with allergies as it strengthens the immune system.

Name: Bee Propolis

Nutrient Content: Rich in 16 amino acids and is a plentiful source of bioflavonoids, which have anti-inflammatory properties, while amino acids play an important role in maintaining a healthy immune system.

Action and Uses: Anti-inflammatory, antimicrobial, antibacterial, antiviral and antifungal properties . Antibacterial, as a salve good for abrasions and bruises. Aids against inflammation of the mucous membranes of the mouth and throat, dry cough and throat, halitosis, tonsillitis, ulcers, and acne. Stimulates immune system.

Name: Probiotics

Nutrient Content: The probiotics most often used as supplements
                       are acidophilus and bifidobacteria.

Action and Uses: These are beneficial bacteria normally present
                       in the digestive tract. They are vital for proper
                       digestion, preventing overgrowth of yeast and
                       pathogens, synthesizing vitamin K.

Comments: Cultured, or fermented, foods also contain
                       various types and amounts of beneficial
                       bacteria. These foods include buttermilk,
                       cheese, airani (kefir), miso, sauerkraut,
                       tempeh, umemboshi plums , and goat's
                       yoghurt.

Name: Chlorella

Nutrient Content: Packed with antioxidants, carotenoids, RNA
                       and DNA nucleic acids, protein, vitamins,
                       minerals and other nutrients.

Action and Uses: Aids the body in the breakdown and
                       elimination of heavy metals and other toxins.

Comments: It is known as the anti-aging green food.

Name: Fish Oil

Nutrient Content: Omega - 3

Action and Uses: Improve skin & hair, reduce blood pressure,
                       aid in prevention of arthritis, lower
                       cholesterol, and triglyceride levels, reduce risk
                       of blood clot formation, beneficial for

cardiovascular disease, eczema, psoriasis, normal development and function of brain.

Comments: Found in sardines, salmon, flaxseed oil, walnut oil, mackerel, cod, menhaden and herrings. A good Norwegian salmon oil is recommended from Carlson Laboratories. Beware of cheap "big box store- pharmacy" brands of fish oil, as they are often loaded with dangerous chemicals.

Name: Flax seed oil

Nutrient Content: Omega-3, magnesium, potassium, fiber, B Vitamins, protein and zinc.

Action and Uses: Reduce pain, inflammation, swelling in arthritis, lower blood cholesterol, lower triglycerides, help reduce hardening effects of cholesterol on cell membranes.

Name: Grape seed oil

Nutrient Content: High source of linolenic acid, lowest in saturated fats. It contains no cholesterol and no sodium. Unlike most oils, it can be heated to high temperatures without producing dangerous and possibly carcinogenic free radicals. This makes it good for use in cooking.

Action and Uses: Grape seed oil contains polyphenols, which are antioxidants. Polyphenols can help slow the process of aging, as well as having anti inflammatory and anti oxidant properties, which also makes it great for helping clear up acne.

Comments: Buy only grape seed oil that is cold-pressed and contains no preservatives.

Name: Moringa Oleifera

Nutrient Content: It is According to the USDA, one cup of fresh, chopped moringa leaves contains two grams of protein, vitamin B6, vitamin C, iron, vitamin B2, vitamin A, and magnesium. Compared to kale; moringa powder can have twice the amount of <u>protein,</u> four times more calcium, six times more iron, 1.5 times more fiber, 97 times more B2, and five times more B3.

Action and Uses: Consuming moringa may actually help you lose weight by boosting your metabolism due to its high levels <u>of B vitamins</u>. B vitamins act as co-enzymes, so they help foster a more efficient metabolism. A more efficient metabolism burns more calories, which can in turn help with weight loss.

Comments: Moringa comes packaged in a few different ways. It is in powder form, as teas, smoothie mixes or as an oil which can be used on the body.
The other most accessible form is moringa leaf powder. Research shows extracts from this part of the plant exhibit the greatest antioxidant activity. The best way to add moringa powder into your diet is by adding it into your smoothies.

Name: Primrose Oil

Nutrient Content: Contains 9 to 10 % gamma-linolenic acid (GLA).

Action and Uses: This fatty acid is known to help prevent hardening of the arteries, heart disease, premenstrual syndrome, multiple sclerosis, high blood pressure. It relieves pain and inflammation, enhances the release of sex hormones, including estrogen and testosterone, aids in lowering cholesterol levels and is beneficial for cirrhosis of the liver. It relieves hot flashes in menopausal women.

Comments: NOTE: Because it promotes the production of estrogen, women suffering from breast cancer that is diagnosed as estrogen-receptor positive (estrogen related) should avoid taking primrose oil. Black currant seed oil is a good substitute.

Name: Spirulina

Nutrient Content: It is unusual in that it is high in protein, which is alkaline forming in the body rather than acid-forming. Spirulina is also rich in vitamins E, B12, C, B1, B5, and B6 as well as beta-carotene, and the minerals zinc, copper, manganese and selenium. It also contains good levels of anti-aging anti-oxidants and of phycocyanin – a blue pigment structurally similar to beta-carotene.

Action and Uses: Spirulina is probably the single most important nutritional supplement you can use to support high level health. Aids in detoxifying the body, helps the body deal with high levels of stress.

Comments: Good quality Spirulina is grown in Hawaii.

Name: Wheatgrass

Nutrient Content: Is known to be highly nutritious. It contains Vitamin A, B12, C, E, B17, folic acid, calcium, potassium, iron, sodium, zinc, magnesium, selenium, phosphorous, copper, sulfur, iodine, manganese, and many other enzymes, carotenoids, and phytonutrients.

Action and Uses:

- Defeats nutritional deficiencies
- Strengthens immune system
- Resolves digestion related problems such as constipation, acidity, piles, colitis, ulcers, diabetes, kidney malfunction, etc
- Combats foul odours of breath and sweat
- Weight loss
- Promotes health and healing
- Beneficial supplement for people suffering from diseases such as cancer, blood pressure, menstrual problems, leukemia, arthritis, insomnia, asthma.

Comments: A good all round supplement

Name: Chaga Mushroom

Nutrient Content: Very high in SOD – antioxidant

Action and Uses: Immune enhancing properties, a tonic,
                          blood purifier, and pain reliever, as
                          well as for tuberculosis, stomachache,
                          ulcers, gastritis, heart or liver disease,
                          worms, and as an internal and external
                          cleanser, called 'soap water'.
                          Colonics of Chaga decoction are used
                          to treat the lower bowel.

Comments: Anti-cancer, anti-tumour.

There is a great deal of evidence to suggest that many of today's diseases may be related to mineral deficiencies.

Here are some examples:

Heart Problems: There is a strong association between magnesium deficiency and heart attack risk.

Immunity: deficiencies of iron, zinc, magnesium and selenium suppress immunity.

Other associations have been made with the following (to name a few).

Infertility: calcium, zinc, selenium, chromium, copper.

Arthritis: copper, calcium, magnesium, potassium, lithium

Cancer: selenium, germanium.

Liver dysfunction: cobalt, selenium, copper, zinc.

Note: Minerals work in conjunction with other minerals. Therefore a combination is the best choice.

Tasks for This Week:

1. Add in a wholefood supplement or two to your health regime.
2. Please note, that there are many other natural supplements available. Research and find your own which may be an appropriate addition to your health regime.

7 WEEK SEVEN

Get Your Body in Shape

Movement

Everything in our bodies is constantly in motion. Blood is circulated around our body by our heart which pumps it, lungs expand and contract while we breathe, eyes scan, and eardrums vibrate. To be alive is to be moving. Prevent movement and you create illness. No movement at all and you are dead. Allow it fully and you achieve wellness.

A body which moves is a body "taking shape." Regular exercise can firm muscles, shed pounds, and add a healthy glow to your complexion. Loving how you feel and how you look are among the rewards.

Keeping to a regular program of exercise is a statement of personal power. It says that you are in control of your own life, that you have endurance, strength, and flexibility. You witness yourself as the chooser, the mover, the changer.

What you do in your body, you can do in your work, your relationships, your dreams, your world at large.

The moving body is the body releasing stress and letting go of pent-up emotions.

Exercise

Exercise doesn't just promote an increase in physical fitness, people who exercise regularly can enjoy a range of secondary benefits. Regular exercise improves sleep, reduces headaches, improves concentration and increases stamina.

Endorphins are released into the brain during exercise and those chemicals promote a sense of positiveness and happiness that will last for some time after the activity. This is an active tool in the fight against depression and a vital move in the preparation for a relaxed life.

Exercise is the distribution process of our nourishment. It aids the assimilation, utilization, and elimination of foods. Moving every joint every day will maintain flexibility and function. We also want to be active enough to keep toned muscles and a toned heart.

Exercise is also very important for immune function. Regular activity increases the circulation of nutrients and the cellular immune components. Also keep in mind that muscle activity is necessary to circulate our lymph fluid.

People are often accused of putting too much time into their careers or families and strenuous physical activity is a great antidote to that. In today's society there is a general emphasis on sedentary lifestyles, and it is a trend that shows little sign of slowing down. This makes it difficult to find an appropriate outlet for mental negativity and accumulated physical frustration.

Physical exertion is great for releasing the toxic emotions that threaten a relaxed sense of wellbeing. You can thrash out tension, anger, frustration and aggression, exercising your mental muscles along with your physical ones.

Exercise, is a personal thing. You probably won't like all forms of activity.

Choose activities according to your individual personality, physical capabilities and the time you have available.

Realistically tailoring your activity to your lifestyle is the best way to ensure that you stick to your exercise regime.

Skilled sports such as skiing or golf are obviously more appealing if you have the time to invest in learning the game and developing your ability to a certain level.

Highly competitive sports should be viewed with caution if you already have an exceptionally stressful lifestyle. Most experts would advise some form of noncompetitive exercise, like swimming, weight-training or walking, for those with limited time and resources. Even as little as twenty minutes a day put aside for such activities will be of great benefit.

A combination of resistance training and aerobic training is best. Resistance training improves metabolism, increases strength, mobility and balance, and also lowers body fat. Aerobic training improves cardiovascular (heart and lungs) functions.

Aerobic activities include swimming, long distance running, cycling, rowing, cross-country skiing and even walking – if it is brisk enough.

Exercise and Weight-Loss

Few weight-loss programs are effective without increasing physical activity. To lose weight or mass, we need to reduce intake and increase output.

Reducing fat stores and adding muscle improves energy utilization by using more calories for active metabolic tissues. Exercise also improves general metabolism and vitality and lowers that important "set point" allowing us to maintain lower weight and body fat with the same food intake.

At a good level of exercise, the body will burn more calories than usual, even 12 hours afterward. Regular exercise is clearly needed to keep fat off.

Daily exercise is essential. If we are just starting out, we should first begin slowly and build to a regular daily program. If we make it a habit, we will really see the benefit. Then, at most we might skip it for one day a week, but only if we must, and then we should stretch and walk anyway. Some aerobics activity is ideal, even 20 – 30 minutes a day, five or six days a week. Our body stores energy, not as calories, but mainly as fat.

Aerobic-type exercises will burn and reduce fat stores, without reducing muscle tissue (weight-loss programs without exercise can cause muscle loss). One to two hours daily of activity as we get into shape.

A 30-minute walk about a half hour after meals is just the thing to further help digestion and assimilation.

Walking Works Wonders

Put the fun factor back into exercise and get your friends to join in. The cheapest, easiest way to get fit lies right at your feet. So take a deep breath, put away the car keys, and step out for the good of your health. It's an exercise routine you can stick to. Imagine a workout that gives you strong, toned muscles without ever setting foot inside a gym, and great abs without doing a single sit-up. You really can get leaner, fitter and sexier just by legging it. And thanks to its "anytime, anyplace," flexibility, walking can slot easily into your life which means it's easy (and cheap) to stick with.

The Plan

This weekly programme contains five "walkouts". Pick and mix between 3 and 5 sessions a week, depending on your level of fitness. You may have at least 2 days rest if you need them. If you're very unfit, or not used to walking briskly, start with three 10-minute sessions per week, and gradually build up.

Walkout 1
Fitness walk, 15 to 20 minutes. Walk at a comfortable pace for five minutes, then gradually increase the speed by seven to ten steps a minute (see "How fast should I be walking ?"). Slow down to a comfortable pace for the last five minutes.

Walkout 2
Hill session, about 30 minutes. Walk at a comfortable pace for 10 minutes to warm up. Increase the pace for 20 seconds, walking uphill. Slow down for a minute or so, then speed up again for another 20 seconds. Repeat eight times. Do a 10-minute cool down, walking at a comfortable pace.

Variation: If there are no hills near you that are long enough, or if you're just starting out and want to take it a bit easier, walk briskly up your chosen slope and then back down to the starting point. Repeat as above.

Walkout 3
Fitness walk, 20 minutes. Same as workout 1.
You can increase the intensity by picking out a person in the distance and aiming to catch up with them, or walking with someone whose strides are longer than yours.

Walkout 4
Interval session, about 30 minutes. Warm up for 10 minutes by walking at a comfortable pace. Then increase your speed for about 50m (or, say, the distance between two street lamps or two trees on your route). Slow back down to starting pace for 100m. Repeat this nine times, then finish with a 10-minute cool-down walk.

Bonus: Interval training increases your overall speed because it builds stamina and endurance.

Walkout 5
Tempo training, 20 minutes. Walk at a comfortable pace for 10 minutes to warm up, then slightly increase the pace for five minutes.
Bonus: Tempo training burns extra calories and helps build stamina, strength and speed.

Walkout 6

Tempo training 50 minutes. Walk at a comfortable pace for 5 minutes to warm up, and then you will walk for 4 minutes and light jog for 1 minute. Repeat this set 7 times. To cool down walk for 5 minutes.

How Fast Should I Be Walking?

Start by walking slowly; at about 5km/h. Gradually increase the pace to 5,5km/h, or more when you're doing intervals or tempo training. Monitor your speed by counting steps: 120 steps per minute is about 5km/h: 135 steps per minute is roughly 6,5km/h (for a real kilojule burn); and 150 steps is about 7-8km/h (serious speed). Rather than counting for a whole minute, count the paces you take in 20 seconds and multiply by three to calculate steps per minute.

When you increase your pace from 5 – 7 km/h, you blast 50% more kilojoules. That means a 65kg woman increasing her speed this way could burn 800kj in half an hour, instead of 550kj.

Walk Right

When you walk with proper form, all your key muscle groups benefit: Here's how:

- Keep your chin lifted. Looking down slows your pace and potentially strains your neck.

- Focus on landing on your heel, then rolling through the ball of the foot to finish with a quick push off the toes. This optimizes speed, too.

- Keep your elbows in and bend your arms at about 90 degrees: they'll swing faster and allow for a quicker pace than extended arms.
- You can add variety and intensity with lunges. Placing your hands on your hips for balance, take a large step forward with

the right leg, lunging until the right knee is bent 90 degrees. Hold for two seconds. Bring left foot to meet right, then step left foot forward into a lunge. Do walking lunges for 1 minute.

With more exercise, our vitality, endurance, and ability to handle stress and life all improve. Try It !

Tasks for This Week:

1. Add in at least 30 minutes of aerobic exercise a day. A brisk walk is splendid exercise and can be done almost anywhere.

2. Important note: Exercise is most beneficial early in the day, shortly after you wake up. Research shows that the effect of morning exercise increases the metabolic rate for about 10 to 12 hours afterwards. If you exercise in the evening, your metabolism will increase for no more than four or five hours, then it will slow down when you go to bed.

8 WEEK EIGHT

Detox Your World

Although I am generally an optimistic person, thinking about chemical pollution of our beautiful planet makes me sad.

There are so many new substances, some highly toxic in nature, which are proving difficult for both Earth and our bodies to handle. We do not have the enzymes to metabolize them.

Our societies' leaders and developers would like us to believe that exposure to tiny amounts of toxic materials poses little or no risk. The hidden danger is in the repeated small exposures over time with regular use. Partly because many chemicals do not break down and accumulate in our bodies. Their presence in the body can cause repeated insults or lead to chronic diseases. Nature does not provide the enzymes necessary to break down all of these synthetic chemicals, nor can our body readily metabolize and excrete them. As the Earth becomes more and more polluted, so do our bodies.

Today's most common diseases are environmental in nature, involving our interaction with our surroundings – contact with viruses, bacteria, fungi, and other parasites, food intake, and exposure to chemicals and wastes in the air and water. These exposures can occur at home, at work, while traveling or shopping, or on vacation.

Our greatest concern individually and as a species regarding environmental chemical contamination is cancer.

The carcinogenicity of many chemicals is well documented. There are many other cancer-causing chemicals that have not been confirmed by research studies. Cancer is the worst possible outcome, but chemical exposure may also result in weakened immune function with increased susceptibility to germs and allergens, disruption of cell integrity and possible changes in DNA, and ultimately, increased sensitivity to other chemicals in the environment. Cancer itself is, in part, the inability of our body to process chemical agents that have carcinogenic potential to cells and tissues.

How Chemicals Cause Damage

Industrial chemicals both contaminate and interact with life. Some can even destroy life when they become concentrated enough. Many pesticides, fungicides, herbicides, and preservative chemicals can cause liver disease, cancer and death. Radioactive fallout and air pollution also affects us.

Industrial and agricultural chemicals that contaminate our soil, our water, and our food are our greatest concerns.
There are two levels to the process whereby chemicals cause disease, particularly cancer.

The first is by direct irritation, causing change at the cellular and DNA level. A chemical that is a potential carcinogen may actually bind to the DNA in the cell nucleus and / or in the mitochondria, thereby altering its structure and potential for normal duplication. It may also make the DNA more vulnerable to the same or other carcinogens. Further generations of the cell with damaged or transmuted DNA may be either metaplastic or malignant. Our bodies have remarkable capabilities when it comes to the repair and even elimination of any abnormal DNA and malignant cells, however, when our immune system is weakened, or there are just too many chemical insults for our body to handle, a chronic inflammation and cancer may develop. Cancer, or malignancy, is a mass of rapidly dividing, undifferentiated cells that takes the body's energy without using it creatively.

Chemical damage is largely due to the generation of free radicals, unstable molecules that can cause irritation and breakdown of tissues unless they are countered by antioxidants in our body.

The antioxidant system is a series of enzymes and essential nutrients within the body that protects us from these chemically-induced free radicals, just as a fine-mesh screen protects us and our home from the shooting sparks generated by burning wood in the fireplace.

Free radicals are a normal product of metabolism; in the body they are generated by both enzymatic and chemical reactions, including the metabolism of fats. Peroxides, epoxides, and superoxides are examples of free radicals. The glutathione peroxidase and superoxidase dismutase enzyme systems neutralize some of these potentially damaging free-radical molecules. Vitamin A and beta-carotene, vitamins C and E, glutathione, and selenium are all important antioxidants that help protect us from disease. Chemical sensitivity and food allergies often go hand in hand as many chemicals are present in food as both additives and contaminants.

Contaminants accidentally get into food as residues of fertilizers, pesticides, or pollutants in the water or air. Additives are deliberately "added" to food, both in processing as ingredients to improve flavor, colour or shelf life.

In our culture, it is possible that indoor chemical pollution is an even bigger concern. Some estimates suggest that pollution is 5 – 10 times more damaging indoors than outdoors. This is because there are so many sources of it – gas heaters and ranges, insulation, carpets and carpet padding, adhesives, aerosols, such as hair sprays and deodorants, insect sprays, pesticide powders, and pest strips, synthetic carpets, drapes, and clothes, cleaning compounds, detergents, deodorizers, and disinfectants, and cosmetics, perfumes, and colognes – to name a few. If we want to reduce chemical exposure, the home is a good place to begin.

Chemicals in Foods

The food industry uses about 3,000 different food additives in a wide variety of packaged and preserved foods. These range from added vitamins and minerals to emulsifiers, buffers, natural and artificial flavouring and colouring, and large amounts of salt and sugar.

Besides the acknowledged additives, there are about 12,000 other chemicals that contaminate our food during the various stages of propagation, growth, harvesting, packing, shipping, and preparation. These chemicals include sprays and pesticides, many of which are more dangerous than most food additives. Plastics are another example of contamination. Plastic wrap contains polyvinyl chloride (PVC), a potentially carcinogenic chemical.

I believe that we should do everything in our personal power to avoid or minimize the use of chemicals and processed foods. Cultivating and consuming wholesome, natural, and organic foods, ideally grown locally and eaten fresh, has long-range benefits for our environment, our bodies, and our health.

People consuming chemicalised foods take a risk. The chemical companies and the food processors make a lot of money, at our expense, both in terms of our health care costs as well as money spent on their products. The health of our planet earth is also at stake. It is in our personal health interest to avoid chemical additives and processed foods, and to eat naturally.

However, even in natural foods such as fruits, vegetables and grains, there is a great deal of potential contamination when these foods and the land on which they are grown are chemically treated. For this reason, we can try to eat organic. Even organic foods can have small amounts of unavoidable environmental contamination, such as rain, contaminated water, chemical residue in soil, and nuclear fallout.

Chemicals in Our Air

Air pollution is of greater concern in regard to general health. There are higher levels of chemical irritants in the air in smoggy, heavily populated, or industrial areas.
Indoor pollution at work, home, in shops, or at hair salons may be much worse than outdoor air pollution because there is more contamination with less dilution.

Chemicals in Water

Water is probably our biggest area of concern in regard to chemical pollution. According to the book The Nontoxic Home (Tarcher, 1986), written by Debra Lynn Dadd. Water-contaminating substances are categorized in the following manner:

1. **Microorganisms:** such as bacteria and viruses is one form of contamination. (Chlorine is usually added to water to reduce these organisms.

2. **Dissolved solids:** These are materials that dissolve in the water, many of which come from the soil. Included in this group are the nitrates, the sulfates, fluoride, and various mineral salts.

3. **Particulates:** un-dissolved materials such as dirt, rust, asbestos or heavy metals – lead, mercury, cadmium, silver, aluminium, cobalt and so, on.

4. **Volatile Chemicals:** Many of these are unsafe even in small amounts. These include pesticides, such as DDT and lindane, chlorinated hydrocarbons, chloroform and other THMs, trichloroethylene (TCE), and many more. Chemical water pollutants include both inorganic and organic substances.

Water Filters

It is also worthwhile and fairly expensive to use a home filter system to protect yourself and your family. Most are reasonably priced and will remove most of the chemical contamination. Solid carbon block filtration is a good basic system, avoid granulated carbon filters. Reverse osmosis filters are also a good choice, however, these systems usually have three different filters and are usually more expensive. Reverse osmosis also needs good water pressure and can waste water.

Bottled water is usually free of toxic chemicals, but it too can come from contaminated groundwater. Polyethylene, a soft plastic commonly used for water containers, can contaminate water, though the level of this toxicity is low.

Drinking tap water is not recommended. Public water treatment leaves much to be desired. Chlorine has become a panacea to treat and prevent microbial contamination. Although such treatment has helped clean up our water, chlorine can interact with organic wastes, such as dead leaves, and form the carcinogenic trihalomethane (THM) chemicals.

Chloroform is commonly found in city waters. In 1979, the EPA set the limit for THMs to be 100 parts per billion (ppb) in water. They estimated that this level would add only 200 cancer deaths per year. Several studies have shown an increased incidence of cancer, especially of the gastrointestinal tract and rectum, in people who drink chlorinated water.

Other problems associated with tap water are that plastic pipes more easily leak or interact with industrial solvents, pesticides, or gasoline. Polyvinyl chloride (PVC), polybutylene (PB), and polyethylene (PE) are three common pipe plastics; the first two are mild carcinogens. Lead and copper pipes also add to contamination of drinking water.

Food Cultivation

Most of the chemical contamination that gets into our foods comes from pesticide sprays used during the sub-classifications of pesticides. The three main classes of chemical pesticides are organochlorides, organophosphates, and carbamates.
Many chemical sprays are used on cultivated vegetables. Cruciferous vegetables may be the biggest problem because they absorb the chemicals so well. Cabbage, broccoli, cauliflower, and Brussels sprouts may be eaten more now because of their alleged reduction of cancer potential, but if they are sprayed with subtle carcinogens, that potential may actually be increased. In this case it may be best to eat organically grown cruciferous vegetables.

Chemicals in Food

There are currently about 3,000 food additives approved for use in the foods we eat or the beverages we drink.

Common Foods That Contain Artificial Flavours

Alcoholic beverages, Baked Goods, Candy, Cereals, Cordials, Desserts, Gelatins, Gum, Ice-cream, Ices, Jams, Jellies, Liquors, Maple syrup, Margarine, Meats, Puddings, Sauces, Seasonings, Shortening, Soda Pop, Soups, Spices, Syrups, Yoghurts.

What is our best approach to food additives ?

First, we should eat more wholesome foods, such as fresh fruits and vegetables, whole grains, nuts, seeds, beans, and range-fed animals. It is also very important to buy and eat less of the packaged foods that contain additives. We should definitely avoid the nitrates and nitrites, as they can form carcinogenic nitrosamines in the food and in our body. The sulfites, such as sulfur dioxide, sodium sulfite, bisulfate, and metabisulfite which are commonly used to prevent or reduce spoilage or discolouration, are best avoided, particularly by people with allergies. BHA and BHT, as well as EDTA, should be consumed minimally as should the flavour enhancer MSG (Monosodium glutamate). Artificial colours and flavours should definitely be left out of our diet.

Food Additives Guide

Additives to Avoid

Artificial colours (FD&C colours)
Sodium nitrite and nitrate
BHT (butylated hydroxytoluene)
Saccharin
Sulfites (especially sodium bisulfate)
Sulfur dioxide
BVO (Brominated Vegetable Oil)

Additives to Limit (use with caution)

BHA (butylated hydroxyanisole)
MSG (monosodium glutamate)
Sugars (sucrose, dextrose, corn syrup)
Artificial flavorings
THBQ
Propyl gallate
EDTA
Hydrogenated vegetable oils
Salt
Aspartame
Caffeine
Propylene glycol
Gums
Xylitol
Aluminium salts

Probably Safe Additives

Vitamins A, C, and E
Beta-carotene or Carotene
Carrageenan
Annatto
Acids – citric, sorbic, lactic
Alginates
Minerals – iron, zinc, and others
Glycerin – mono- and diglycerides
Gelatin
Pectin
Natural flavoring
Calcium proprionate
Polysorbate 60, 65, 80
Sorbitol
Sodium benzoate
Lecithin
Casein and lactose
Vanillin
Potassium sorbate

Pollutants in the Home

Most of us are exposed to more chemicals in the home than anywhere else, mainly because there are so many possible uses for chemicals and also because we spend more of our time in our own or friend's homes.

Regular contact with various chemicals weakens us immunologically and makes us more susceptible to disease in general.

Most cleaning supplies, cosmetics, and toiletries have a dual route to irritation and toxicity – by contact and by inhalation of the fumes. If ingested, most of these products may be very dangerous, even deadly.

There are many products available which are less toxic or nontoxic. Safe cleaners, for example, include lemon, baking soda, vinegar, salt, and trisodium phosphate. Check at local health food shops for safer products.

Home Cleaning Supplies

Detergents – may cause eye irritation
Fabric softeners – residues on clothes can be irritating or allergenic
Spray Starch – phenol, formaldehyde (aerosol)
Mothballs – paradichlorobenzene – toxic to the liver and kidney, irritating to mucous membranes.
Dry cleaning spot removers – perchloroethylene – a solvent that when inhaled can irritate the liver and nervous system.
Chlorine Bleach – should not be mixed with ammonia or vinegar, as the resulting chloramines can be toxic fumes.
Ammonia – may cause rash or irritate eyes and skin, especially in aerosols.
Drain cleaners – lye, caustic sodium hydroxide – very toxic to skin and when ingested.
Oven cleaner – lye aerosols are the most dangerous
Furniture, and floor polish – nitrobenzene, naphthalene, and phenols.

Silver polish – ammonia, petroleum products
Glass cleaners – ammonia, blue dye – aerosols worse than spray pumps.
Air fresheners – phenol, cresol, ethanol, xylene
Germ-killing disinfectants – cresol, phenol, ethanol, formaldehyde – irritating, especially to eyes.
Carpet shampoo and upholstery cleaner – perchloroethylene, ethanol, ammonia, detergents.
Dishwasher detergents – chlorine, detergents – should not be mixed with ammonia or ingested.

Toiletries

Toothpaste – phenol, cresol, ethanol, artificial colour and flavor.
Mouthwash- hydrogen peroxide, phenol, cresol, ethanol, ammonia, formaldehyde, artificial colour and flavor.
Cosmetics and mascara – polyvinylpyrrolidine plastic (PVP), artificial colours, plastic resins, alcohol formaldehyde.
Talcum Powder – may contain asbestos
Perfume and aftershave – alcohol, phenol, cresol, trichloroethylene, formaldehyde, artificial colours and fragrance.
Aerosol hairspray – PVP, formaldehyde, artificial colour and fragrance.
Antiperspirants and deodorants – aluminium chlorohydrate, ammonia, alcohol, formaldehyde, artificial fragrance.
Dandruff shampoo – PVP, formaldehyde, detergents, artificial colours and fragrance.
Hair colour – coal tar, dyes, ammonia, detergents.
Hair removers – ammonium thioglycolate.
Bubble bath – detergent, artificial colour and fragrance
Nail polish and remover – acetone, phenol, toluene, xylene.
Denture cleaners – many salts with artificial colours, fragrance, and preservatives.
Disposable diapers – synthetic fibers, various deodorizing chemicals
Spermicides – methylbenzethonium (benzene) chloride, alcohol, formaldehyde, perfumes, preservatives.

Feminine douches and sprays – ammonia, phenol, detergents, artificial fragrance, talc (may contain asbestos).

Clothes

Permanent Press – resins, formaldehyde

Fabric dyes – dichlorobenzene, benzidine

Flame-resistant fabrics – TRIS – now banned in children's sleepwear because of carcinogenicity.

Synthetic fibers – nylon, polyester, acrylic – which are all plastics.

Art and Home Office Supplies

Glues – epoxy contains vinyl chloride, formaldehyde, and ethanol; "super glue" has acrylonitrile, phenol, naphthalene – all are toxic.

Permanent ink markers – acetone, toluene, xylene, ethanol, cresol

Typewriter correction fluid – cresol, trichloroethylene, naphthalene, ethanol

Computer terminals - may cause eye irritation, headache, fatigue, and neck, shoulder, and back pains.

Television – may cause eye irritation, headache, fatigue.

Plastics

Polyurethane foam – beds, cushions, pillows – lung, skin and eye irritants.

Polyester – clothing, bedding, diapers, tampons, upholstery – may cause irritation, allergy, skin rash.

Nylon – clothing, toothbrushes, other brushes, upholstery and carpets, and so on (probably safe).

Acrylics – made from acrylonitriles – acrylic fiber, waxes, paint, plexiglass.

Polyethylene – containers, wrappers, kitchenware, plastic bags, squeeze bottles – possibly carcinogenic.

Vinyl chloride – worst of the plastics – carcinogenic

Polyvinyl chloride – adhesives, containers, records, tapes, toys, beach balls, pacifiers, raincoats, boots – can release vinyl chloride, which can cause cancer, liver disease, birth defects, and more.

Urea-formaldehyde plastic resins – particleboard, plywood, insulation, tissues and towels – outgas formaldehyde, a suspected carcinogen.

Fluorocarbon plastic – tetrafluoroethylene – Teflon, nonstick coating, ironing board covers, irritant to skin, eyes, respiratory tract.

Other Home Toxins

Smoke – 96 per cent of cigarette smoke pollutes the air and increases carbon monoxide levels. It is also an irritant and secondary smoking is becoming more of a concern.

Garbage – can bring insects and rodents. Keep the house clean and recycle wastes.

Gas appliances – emit gas fumes, carbon monoxide.

Kerosene lamps and heaters – kerosene fumes, carbon monoxide.

Fireplaces and wood stoves – emit chemicals in wood, carbon monoxide

Particleboard – urea- formaldehyde – possibly carcinogenic.

Foam insulation – urea-formaldehyde foam insulator (UFFI) – carcinogenic, banned in 1982 but later re approved.

Home Pesticides

These range from mildly dangerous to very dangerous.

Rodent killers – mousetraps, arsenic, strychnine, phosphorous – deadly if eaten.

Insecticides – all kinds, for various bugs. Pyrethrum, a plant extract, is useful. Most other chemicals, even "inert ingredients," may be dangerous.

Lice shampoos – lindane (Kwell) – when used on body, may be carcinogenic. They are used for lice and crabs and also an insecticide. Pyrethrin powders and sprays may be helpful; useful for animals too, but not for humans.

Suggestions for Reducing Waste and Use of Toxic Products

1. Avoid aerosol sprays, such as deodorants, hairsprays, and cleaners.
2. Avoid plastic containers or use products with comparably minimal waste, for example bulk cheese instead of individually wrapped slices.
3. Use Biodegradable products, such as paper, not plastic, water based soaps, eggs packed in cardboard, products, waxed paper rather than plastic wrap.
4. Purchase reusable products, such as cloth napkins, towels, returnable bottles, rechargeable batteries.
5. Recycle everything possible, such as glass, cans, paper, cardboard, plastics.
6. Avoid chlorofluorocarbon (CFO) products, such as polystyrene (Styrofoam) containers and packaging protectors, whose   production and breakdown are polluting the atmosphere and destroying the ozone layer.
7. Reuse as much as possible, such as paper bags, plastic bags, cardboard boxes, bottles, Styrofoam packing pellets.
8. Buy more durable products.
9. Buy less whenever possible.
10. Shop at farmer's markets where products are available in bulk, where there is less fancy and costly packaging, and they support using recycled plastic and paper bags.
11. Use natural, organic toiletries without any chemicals.

Health Tips

1. Minimise the purchase of plastics, Styrofoam, and other non-biodegradable products. Pre-cycle means not buying products you cannot recycle. This will create a demand for the production of environmentally sound packaging.
2. Avoid processed foods, particularly those that contain highly refined ingredients.
3. Reduce or eliminate food additives, particularly preservatives, artificial flavours, and artificial sweeteners.

4. Additives to avoid include the artificial colours, excess sugars, and salt, BHA and BHT, nitrites and sulfites.
5. A shopping guideline to follow is: "If you can't pronounce it, don't buy it."
6. Buy and use organic foods, those that are grown without chemical fertilizers and pesticides; this action supports the organic food industry and the consciousness of cleaner food. Much produce is contaminated with fumigants and fungicides even after it has been harvested. Organic food items are usually found at health food shops.
7. Buy organic cruciferous vegetables (i.e. cabbage, broccoli, Brussels sprouts, cauliflower) if they are heavily sprayed in your country.
8. Avoid aluminium and Teflon cookware; use glass, Pyrex, iron or stainless steel.
9. Minimize overall use of drugs, particularly over-the-counter drugs and unnecessary prescription drugs.
10. Reduce use of carcinogenic drugs, such as the anti-parasitic drugs lindane (Kwell) and metronidazole (Flagyl), estrogens, and the antifungal griseofulvin.
11. Avoid using aerosols, artificial scents, and toilet colourings. Use herbs and naturally fragrant oils instead.
12. Research and invest in a water filter for your home.
13. Try natural drain cleaners, such as hot water with vinegar or baking soda.
14. Avoid tobacco smoke around you.
15. Avoid living near toxic industry, such as chemical plants, refineries, toxic dump sites, or water-treatment plants.
16. Avoid living near power lines and electrical plants, and any excessive electrical exposure, all of which may pose some health risks. Note that our bodies are electromagnetic in nature.
17. Avoid traveling in rush-hour traffic, if possible, or behind buses and trucks to reduce carbon monoxide and hydrogen gas exposure.
18. Obtain natural lighting or full-spectrum lights at work.

9 WEEK NINE

Power Naps

I was so excited when I came across this article story from BBC news. I am a big fan of taking mid-day naps and have been as far back as I can remember.

Whatever the season, whether it falls under a summer siesta, cold winter snooze warmly wrapped up with your favourite blanket, or a scented spring mid day nap… it is worth while indulging in one.

Nap 'Boosts' Brain Learning Power

US scientists claim that a nap during the day improves the brain's ability to absorb new information.

Volunteers who slept for 90 minutes during the day did better at cognitive tests than those who were kept awake. Results of the University of California at Berkeley study involving 39 healthy adults were presented at a conference.

A UK-based sleep expert said it was hard to separate the pure "memory boosting" effects of sleep from those of simply being less tired.

"Sleep not only rights the wrong of prolonged wakefulness, but, at a neurocognitive level, it moves you beyond where you were before you took a nap." - Dr Matthew Walker, UC Berkeley

The wealth of study into the science of sleep in recent years has so far failed to come up with conclusive evidence as to the value of a quick "siesta" during the day.

The latest study suggests that the brain may need sleep to process short-term memories, creating "space" for new facts to be learned.

In their experiment, 39 healthy adults were given a hard learning task in the morning – with broadly similar results, before half of them were sent for their siesta. When the tests were repeated, the nappers outperformed those who had carried on without sleep.

Checks on brain electrical activity suggested that this process might be happening in a sleep phase between deep sleep, and dreaming sleep, called stage 2 non-rapid eye movement sleep, when fact-based memories are moved from "temporary storage" in the brain's hippocampus to another area called the pre-frontal cortex. Brain 'inbox'.

Dr Matthew Walker, who led the study, reported at the AAAS conference in San Diego, said: "Sleep not only rights the wrong of prolonged wakefulness, but, at a neurocognitive level, it moves you beyond where you were before you took a nap. "It's as though the e-mail inbox in your hippocampus is full, and, until you sleep and clear out all those fact e-mails, you're not going to receive any more mail. "It's just going to bounce until you sleep and move it into another folder."

However, Professor Derk-Jan Dijk, the director of the Surrey Sleep Research Centre, said that there was no clear evidence that daytime napping offered a distinct advantage over sleeping just once over 24 hours.

"The sleep-wake cycle is not as rigid as we might think – we have the capability to sleep in different ways." He said that while the brain effect reported in the study might be spotted in a laboratory setting, the picture became more clouded in the "real world". "The size of these effects are much more difficult to assess – if I have to learn something, for example, it's easier to do this when I'm feeling awake and alert than when I'm sleepy."

Benefits

- More energy
- Improve productivity by over 30%
- Improve alertness by up to 100%
- Reduce stress and the risk of heart disease by 34%
- Better negotiation and communication
- Reduce risk of accidents at work and on the road
- Happiness and wellbeing

The Siesta has existed for thousands of years and was previously regarded as a physical necessity rather than a luxury. While the traditional Mediterranean (Greek, Spanish, Italian) style siesta can last for up to two hours to avoid the hottest part of the day, there is actually a biological need for people in all climates to have a short rest in the afternoon to revive energy levels.

The form of rest recommended for health and productivity benefits is a short 10-20 minute nap, and not the 2 hour long siesta normally associated with Mediterranean countries.

Research shows that the majority of people suffer from tiredness twice in every 24 hour period. We are what's called Bi-phasic; we need two periods of sleep; a long one at night and a shorter one during the day. The early afternoon brings a drop in energy levels, not as severe as night time, but sufficient to make it difficult to concentrate and think clearly.

By having a short nap we can help ourselves think more clearly by more productive and reduce the risk of heart disease. Tiredness can also be a cause of accidents.

A short 10-20 minute nap is all that is needed to restore our concentration, alertness and improve productivity for the afternoon.

Famous People Who Napped

- Bill Clinton napped while President of the United States to help him cope with the pressures of office.

- Brahms napped at the piano while he composed his famous lullaby.

- Napoleon napped between battles while sitting on his horse.

- Churchill maintained that he had to nap in order to cope with his wartime responsibilities.

- Geniuses such as Edison and da Vinci napped.

- Margaret Thatcher napped in order to be at her best.

- Einstein napped frequently during the day to help him think more clearly. He would sit in his favourite armchair with a pencil in his hand and purposefully doze off. He would wake when the pencil dropped, ensuring he did not enter a deep sleep from which it would be difficult to wake up.

Biological Need for Naps

In recent years, studies have suggested that we have a biological need for afternoon naps. Contrary to popular belief, eating lunch does not bring on drowsiness, although a heavy lunch, carbohydrates and alcohol can make us more tired.

Our 'biological clock' regulates certain bodily functions such as blood pressure, heart rate, body temperature and hormonal secretions as well as telling us when we need to rest, to maintain health and wellbeing. The Circadian Rhythm regulates daily rhythms in the body. Studies show that there is a strong biological tendency for humans to become tired and possibly fall asleep in the early or mid afternoon as well as at night. It happens about 8 hours after we wake up in the morning. There is a drop in body temperature at this time too which may be more pronounced in men.

The afternoon level of fatigue is not as pronounced as our night time pattern, but sufficient to reduce our effectiveness and performance.

If we do not get enough sleep at night time, then the need for another rest during the day is even greater. However, sleep deficiency in the long term can be a serious problem and medical help should be sought. Occasional late nights and loss of sleep can be recovered at weekends and by short naps, but should not be made a daily pattern. Napping does not make up for serious sleep deficiency.

Research (published 2007) by Harvard School of Public Health in the US and the University of Athens Medical School conducted over a 6 year period with 24,000 men and women have found that a short nap in the early afternoon can reduce the risk of heart disease by 34%.

Warning

However research by the University of Birmingham and from Guangzhou Hospital in China has also shown in a study involving 16,480 people, that those who napped were 26% more at risk of getting Type 2 Diabetes than those who did not nap.

Several factors which may be behind the link included disrupted night-time sleep and an association between napping and reduced physical activity.

Apparently factors like genetics and being overweight are more significant in the possible development of Type 2 diabetes.

Waking up from napping also activates hormones and mechanisms in the body that stop insulin working effectively and this could predispose people to Type 2 Diabetes – which can develop when the insulin the body makes does not work properly. People who are overweight or obese and therefore more at risk of developing Type 2 Diabetes, can have problems sleeping.

In terms of being major risk factors for developing Type 2 diabetes, disturbed sleep or napping are likely to remain less significant than already established risk factors such as being overweight, being over the age of 40 or having a history of diabetes in the family.

Anyone concerned about their health or about developing Diabetes Type 2 should consult their doctor before adopting napping on a regular basis.

Please note that exercise and weight loss is part of the Med Life Diet Program which would reduce the risk of the development of diabetes.

NASA has done studies for astronauts and pilots, to determine what the best sleep patterns are to maintain maximum performance. They discovered that after a short nap there was a 34% improvement in performance and 54% in alertness. Although these tests were performed for astronauts, the benefits would apply equally well to any industry. It is hard to imagine any other method of productivity enhancement having such profound effects.

In 1975 Dr Roger Broughton of the University of Ottawa first proposed that naps were a natural part of the human sleep cycle. He found that, even after a full night's sleep, people have a strong tendency to fall asleep in the early afternoon. When volunteers were put into a time-free environment, they tended to sleep in two time periods; one at night and another about twelve hours later in the early afternoon.

The Circadian Rhythm of the body is actually 25 hours, so the sleep pattern in a time-free environment would get pushed forward an hour each day. We tend to ignore this for reasons of practicality and work routines by regulating our waking time to the same time each day.

The second wave of tiredness happens about 8 hours after we wake up in the morning. So during the early afternoon between 1.30pm and 3.00pm we are likely feel tired again. A short nap of 10-20 minutes can satisfy this desire for sleep and allow us to wake up feeling refreshed and much more alert.

Tests with volunteers have shown that a short nap can restore energy levels so they can take on more tasks, feel more alert and do significantly better in tests of mental performance.

How Long Should The Nap Be ?

The ideal nap should be between 10-20 minutes. Sleep has been found to follow a cycle where we go through five stages or depths of sleep. These are measured by muscle tone, eye movement and the electrical activity of the brain.

Brain waves are measured according to speed with the quickest being Alpha-rhythms followed by the slower Beta-rhythms and the slowest being Theta and Delta. One sleep cycle (which includes all five depths of sleep) lasts around 90 minutes and is repeated 5-6 times each night.

Stage one is the transition from wakefulness to sleep which may last around 5 minutes.

Stage two is characterised by slower breathing and heart rates and will last for up to 30 minutes, after which we enter **stages 3 and 4** which are the deepest levels of sleep.

Stage 5 brings REM and the dream state. To benefit from a short nap it is important that we do not enter the deepest stages of sleep.
We need to wake up before we enter stage 3; otherwise we are likely to find it difficult to wake up again.
When people experience grogginess after napping it is probably because they have over slept.

If they are chronically over tired, they may pass more quickly to stage 3 sleep which will make it difficult to wake up. The short nap is not a replacement for proper night-time sleep.

Anyone suffering from chronic fatigue or difficulty in sleeping at night should consult their doctor. The ideal length of time is between ten and twenty minutes although even two or three minutes can be beneficial.
The use of a timer, mobile phone alarm or a nudge from a friend is encouraged to avoid over-sleeping.

Tasks for This Week:

1. Incorporate a minimum 10 – 20 minute mid-day nap.

10 WEEK TEN

Stress Management

Being well is more than the absence of illness. It is having the energy to do the things you dream of. Wellness is the belief that your body wants to heal itself and that you can improve your health over time, rather than stand by and watch it deteriorate.

Having a healthy body prevents chronic, degenerative illnesses that are primarily products of our lifestyle. Wellness demands that we take responsibility for our own health and make changes in the way we live in order to help our body function more optimally. We are required to take action and ask the empowering questions, rather than just accept the cultural norm.

In a health plan, the time to tackle the problem is when you have the first small signs. Paying attention to what your body is trying to tell you is the first step to creating health and wellbeing.

Listening to your body can help you make positive changes in your lifestyle that will affect not only your problem, but your entire well-being. For example, if your indigestion happens when your stress level is high, then you can focus on building stress management tools. If your indigestion happens after you eat milk products, then the solution may be the elimination of dairy products.

Most of us make short-lived attempts towards wellness. We begin a new diet each Monday, make New Year's resolutions that we've forgotten by the end of the month. It's not that we aren't trying, we are. But in order to implement long-lasting changes in lifestyle we need a plan or a lifestyle system to implement.

The following exercise is a great way to discover and prioritise which areas of your life need attention. You may feel that your relationships have little or nothing to do with the fact that you have a constant tummy ache, but until you sort them out, you can't know for sure.

The mind is not separate from the body. It has now been well accepted that the thoughts we have influence our physical condition.

All areas of our lives affect our sense of well-being.

Life Analysis Chart

How satisfied are you today in each of these areas of your life ?

Rate them on a scale from 1 to 10, with 1 being the most dissatisfied to 10 being the most satisfied.

No	Life Areas	Rate
1	Romantic Relationships (husband, wife, girlfriend, boyfriend, fiancé, etc.)	
2	Family Relationships	
3	Social Life	
4	Intellectual stimulation	
5	Exercise	
6	Food and Nutrition	
7	Psychological / Emotional health	
8	Work	
9	Environmental (where you live	

	and work)	
10	Spiritual	
11	Leisure / Hobbies / Play	
12	Sex	

Now look at your results. Take note of the areas of your life with the lowest score. These are the areas of your life which you have paid less attention to recently.

Are you generally satisfied or dissatisfied with your life ? People with 8s, 9s, and 10s generally feel pretty good about themselves; their lives are moving in the right direction.

People with 0s, 1s, 2s, and 3s may be feeling a lack of confidence and have low self-esteem. If you have lots of low scores you may want to boost your support systems. Find a friend to talk to or get a professional counselor to help you sort through your priorities.

Your life analysis chart may change from time to time depending on what goes on in your life at that particular time.

Self Responsibility Means...

- Developing an awareness of your own physical, mental and emotional processes and patterns.

- Discovering and exploring your real needs, and finding ways to meet them directly.

- Recognise and understand that you are unique and know yourself better than anyone else.

- Making choices and living courageously in the midst of uncertainty.

- Creating the life you want, rather than just reacting to whatever comes along.

- Asking simply and directly for what you need and want from others.

- Expressing yourself - both your ideas and feelings in ways that effectively communicate to other people who you are and what you know.

- Respecting your body through healthy eating, a healthy lifestyle and exercise.

- Creating and nurturing close relationships with others.

- Engaging in projects that are meaningful to you, being supportive of others, and respecting your environment.

Work

We use work to give structure to our time and meaning to our lives, to earn our livelihood, to express our talents, our dreams, our creativity, to change ourselves and the world at large. As such, work is both necessary and desirable. But when it becomes hard and serious to the point of causing excessive stress, or depression, or a sense of personal frustration or worthlessness, it undermines both our health and our happiness. That is why we consider work in the context of health and wellbeing.

"Nothing is really work unless you would rather be doing something else." - J.M. Barrie

"Pleasure in the job puts perfection in the work." - Aristotle

"Choose a job you love, and you will never have to work a day in your life." - Confucius

Burnout is an all-too-familiar phenomenon in all jobs, at all levels. It happens when people are stuck in jobs they do not like, in jobs that fail to satisfy their needs. Burnout is quite common among those in the helping professions. The "helpers" often turn out to be "rescuers" who take on unnecessary and unrealistic burdens and actually undermine their own health.

Six ways to prevent burnout:

- Self care – through optimum nutrition, exercise and the creation of a supportive environment.

- Take regular deep relaxation and frequent mini-relaxations.

- Awareness of rescuing tendencies, i.e. doing for people what they ought to be doing for themselves.

- Recognise feelings of being a victim and reverse them to feelings of empowerment.

- Directly asking for what you want and need, especially of appreciation and attention.

- Exercise your creativity on a regular basis.

- Acceptance of your limitations - with compassion.

Take one method that appeals to you because you probably need it the most. Focus on that one alone drawing your awareness to it as you go through your day. Your awareness will build the foundation from which change will happen more easily.

Stress, Work Choices, and Alternatives

Stress-reducing activities can transform your attitude towards work and liven up your state of health and emotional wellbeing.

Here are some suggestions that can help you cope with stress and transform your attitudes towards your work:

- Moving and breathing exercises designed to reduce stress such as Tai Chi, yoga, walking in nature.

- Apply positive thinking and creative brainstorming to relieve stressful problems.

- Asserting yourself to make your needs known.

- Breaking typical game-playing patterns in communications.

Applying the principles of health and wellness to working means that you assume full responsibility for yourself and your choices. It means loving and respecting yourself to make the necessary changes.

It is recognizing that you have choices at hand. There are alternatives and other jobs available if need be. There are ways of dealing with stress in your present job. There are ways of transforming your work by incorporating the attitudes that enhance play. There are ways to give up being so serious – to stop being the rescuer for the whole world. There are ways of discovering your real needs and fulfilling them; of discovering your real talents and using them; of discovering your many options and trying them out.

The Planet at Play

Our work and our play can make us realize our reliance on each other as a species, or it can undermine it. Most people desire a form of employment that serves some meaningful purpose, even though in the short run they may function as if they are only in it for personal gain. Work that harms the earth and its resources, work that creates weapons of mass destruction, work that generates greed, jealousy, and fear, and alienates people from one another …. This is work that also harms the worker, in body and inner peace.

If we are to genuinely enjoy the fruits of our labors, we must examine their impact on the planet as a whole, and reaffirm our commitment to letting everybody prosper.

Your Internal Dialogue

You communicate with yourself more than you do with anyone else. Talking to yourself is more formally referred to as intrapersonal communication, and it is sometimes called the internal dialogue, although it is more of a monologue.

These conversations with yourself actually structure your reality since they influence what you find "out there", they will have an impact on your health and happiness. We say "love is blind" not because it diminishes our sight. On the contrary, it usually intensifies it. The blindness refers to the inability to see what you previously considered bad, ugly, or meaningless.

Love causes you to change your outlook on life and subsequently the language you use to describe it. As a result, the world appears to be more beautiful and what's more, you usually feel better too.

If we really understood this connection between language and our reality, then the focus of our attention on health would undergo a radical change.

Instead of talking to ourselves about germs, flu, headaches, arthritis, and senility, we would talk about enthusiasm, strength, balance, energy, and joy. If we appreciated that what we find is really a function of what we look for, our sense of responsibility for our own life and health would increase dramatically.

Self-Talk and Self-Concept

A strong, worthy impression of yourself goes hand in hand with a strong, worthy mind and body. Your health and wellness depends upon your self- perception. These inner conversations, internal dialogues, are you talking to yourself all day long. What once appeared to be someone else's judgment of you now is your own daily judgment, not only of yourself, but most likely of everyone around you.

This is how you furnish the stage on which you act out your personal drama: by constantly judging, endlessly choosing the right category or box in which to safely place each person and situation you encounter. This is a very tiring way of life !

Once you realize how frustrating and exhausting this self-talk is, you can resolve to change it. Try setting aside a few short periods a day in which you simply listen to your inner dialogue.

Write out the dialogue or make a list of the negative messages you continuously hear yourself repeating. It is amazing how predictable and uncreative these messages are.

Firstly notice them, then when you get tired of them, you may be more motivated to try a strategy to turn them off. Some people burst into song, whistle or physical exercise are a good way to turn your attention away from them.

Interpersonal Communication

Interpersonal communication is when you talk to other people. Aiming for total agreement in communication sets you up for failure. You can't win at that game. Aiming for understanding and mutual respect offers the best chance of ensuring that everybody can win.

Any problem big or small, within a family, always seems to start with bad communication. Someone isn't listening.
- Emma Thompson.

In order for us to trust others, we need to be able to trust ourselves. We nourish trust for ourselves by taking responsibility for our own lives and living with integrity, authenticity, love, and compassion.

Some common causes for breakdowns in communication:

- Conversations that are really monologues, and thus do not create real deep two-way sharing.

- Failure to express real feelings, resulting in dishonesty and non-assertiveness.

- Inflexibility, which shows up in absolutes and generalizations.

- Failure to listen.

- Manipulative communication (sometimes called "game playing") – another form of dishonest communication.

Stress

Stress is the 'wear and tear' our minds and bodies experience as we attempt to cope with our continually changing environment.

In the future, stress may come to be seen as the primary contributing cause of most diseases. Research continues to link stress to more and more symptoms and diseases, both acute and chronic.

Stress is the automatic 'fight-or-flight' response in the body, activated by adrenaline and other stress hormones, which stimulate a variety of physiological changes, such as increased heart rate and blood pressure, faster breathing, muscle tension, dilated pupils, dry mouth and increased blood sugar. In simple biological terms, stress is the state of increased arousal necessary for an organism to defend itself when faced with danger.

During times of increased stress our body's nutrients are used more rapidly to meet the increased amounts of many of these functions.

Whenever we feel anxious, tense, tired, frightened, elated or depressed, we are undergoing stress. Few aspects of life are free from the events and pressures that generate such feelings, and stress has become an acceptable and unavoidable part of normal everyday existence.

In fact, contrary to popular assumptions, stressed lifestyles are not an exclusively modern phenomenon – stress has always been intrinsic to human existence, and life without stress would be unbearable.

For example, certain types of stress, such as physical and mental exercise, sex, and intense creativity, are actually very desirable. It is only when real or perceived change overwhelms the body's ability to cope, that stress becomes harmful (distress), leaving us prone to unwanted physical, mental or emotional reactions and illnesses.

Types of Stress

The causes of stress are multiple and varied, but they can be divided into two general categories external and internal:

External Stressors

- Physical environment – noise, bright lights, heat, confined spaces.

- Social interaction – rudeness, bossiness or aggressiveness by others.

- Organizational – rules, regulations, 'red tape', deadlines.

- Major life events – death of a relative, lost job, promotion, new baby.

- Daily hassles – commuting, misplacing keys, mechanical breakdowns.

Internal Stressors

- Lifestyle choices – caffeine, not enough sleep, overloaded schedule.

- Negative self-talk – pessimistic thinking, self-criticism, over-analysing.

- Mind traps – unrealistic expectations, taking things personally, all-or-nothing thinking, exaggerating, rigid thinking.

- Stressful personality traits – type A, perfectionist, workaholic.

These factors generate various symptoms of emotional and mental stress, the most common including: anger, fear, and depression.

Common Stress Factors

- Attitude toward self
- Personal financial state
- Moving
- Traffic tickets
- Tests in school
- Meeting someone new
- Raising children
- Demands at the office
- Job and career challenges
- Promotion, job loss
- Emotional challenges: personal relationships, fear, anger, loneliness
- Family changes: marriage, divorce, separation, a new baby
- Physical challenges: weather changes, extreme climates, athletic events
- Health challenges: illness, injury, surgery, chemical exposures
- Life changes: adolescence, aging, pregnancy, menopause.

Please note, that stress is not from the situations or incidents themselves, rather, *real stress comes from the way we react to them.*

For stress to arise and negatively influence our health, we must experience something as a danger.

When we do, anxiety is generated, which we often experience as fear or a feeling of threat to our survival.

If we view stress positively, we see it as simply a survival response. But if we cannot handle the stress, we may experience the symptoms and diseases of stress.

Learning to adapt our attitude and find suitable outlets for our stress is a very important long-term plan.

Stress produces irritating molecules that generate immunological changes, damage cells, and inflame organ and blood vessel linings. Stress responses also use up more vital nutrients which can lead to deficiencies.

Stress has also been shown to decrease protective antibodies and reduce the important T lymphocytes that function in the cellular immune system. Chronic stress is clearly a culprit in the generation of aging and degenerative diseases.

In addition, stress affects the stomach and pancreas and thus our digestion. Stress initially increases stomach hydrochloric acid production, leading to indigestion, heartburn, gastritis, and ulcer problems.

Stress- Related Symptoms and Diseases

- Fatigue
- Irritability
- Headaches
- Muscle tension
- Neck and Back pains
- Atherosclerosis
- High Blood Pressure

- Diabetes
- Arthritis
- Cancer
- Indigestion
- Diarrhea
- Constipation
- Peptic Ulcer
- Irritable Bowel
- Loss of appetite
- Anorexia Nervosa
- Weight changes
- Insomnia
- Depression
- Infections
- Eczema
- Psoriasis
- Allergies
- Asthma
- Nutritional deficiencies
- Premenstrual symptoms
- Sexual problems
- Psychological problems

Childhood Influences and Upbringing

A traumatic childhood is likely to lead to greater levels of stress as an adult. A difficult childhood is also more likely to lead to low self-esteem, low self-assertiveness, difficulty expressing personal beliefs, attitudes and feelings, and a tendency to depend on others to provide a sense of emotional wellbeing and self-worth.

Over reliance on others is likely to lead to frustration as it is difficult for expectations to be met. This leads to feelings of frustration, anger, depression and hopelessness in adulthood.

Unrealistic Expectations

Unrealistic expectations are a common source of stress. People often become upset about something, not because it is innately stressful but because it does not concur with what they expected. Take, for example, the experience of driving in slow-moving traffic. If it happens at rush hour, you may not like it but it should not surprise or upset you. However, if it occurs on a Sunday afternoon, especially if it makes you late for something, you are more likely to be stressed by it.

When expectations are realistic, life feels more predictable and therefore more manageable. There is an increased feeling of control because you can plan and prepare yourself (physically and psychologically). For example, if you know in advance when you have to work overtime or stay late, you will take it more in your stride than when it is dropped on you at the last minute.

Attitudes and Beliefs

A lot of stress results from our beliefs. We have literally thousands of premises and assumptions about all kinds of things that we hold to be the truth. They can be everything from, 'You can't beat the system' and 'The customer is always right', to 'Men shouldn't show their emotions', and 'Children should tidy their rooms'. We have beliefs about how things are, how people should behave and about ourselves ('I can never remember people's names'). Most of our beliefs are held unconsciously so we are unaware of them. This gives them more power over us and allows them to run our lives.

Beliefs cause stress in two ways. The first is the behaviour that results from them. For example, if you believe that work should come before pleasure, you are likely to work harder and have less leisure time than you would otherwise.

If you believe that people should meet the needs of others before they meet their own, you are likely to neglect yourself to some extent. These beliefs are expressions of a personal philosophy or value system, which results in increased effort and decreased relaxation – a formula for stress. There is no objective truth to begin with. These are really just opinions but they lead to stressful behaviours. Uncovering the unconscious assumptions behind actions can be helpful in changing one's lifestyle.

The second way in which beliefs cause stress is when they are in conflict with those of other people. However, it should always be remembered that personal assumptions are not the truth but rather opinions and, therefore, they can be challenged. In situations of conflict it is always helpful if the protagonists attempt to revise their beliefs, or at least admit that the beliefs held by the other person may be just as valid as their own. This mind-opening exercise usually helps to diminish stressful antagonism.

Stress-Management Techniques

It would not be possible, or desirable, to eliminate all the effects of stress in our lives. The aim of stress management should be to harness and control the effects of stress to help to enrich our physical, mental and emotional well-being. By getting to the root causes of your stress, you can not only relieve current problems and symptoms, but you can also prevent recurrences.

Corrective action falls into three main categories:

- Change your thinking
- Change your behaviour
- Change your lifestyle

Change Your Thinking

Reframing: is one of the most powerful and creative stress reducers. It is a technique used to change the way you perceive things in order to feel better about them. We all do this inadvertently at times. The key to reframing is to recognize that there are many ways to interpret the same situation. It is like the age-old question: Is the glass half empty or half full ? The answer of course is that both or either, depending on your point of view. However, if you see the glass as half full, it will feel different than seeing it as half empty because the way we feel almost always results from the way we think. The bottom line about reframing is this: there are many ways of seeing the same thing, so you might as well pick the version that you like. Reframing does not change the external reality, but simply helps you to view things differently and less stressfully.

Positive Thinking

When faced with stressful situations try to avoid becoming preoccupied with debilitating, gloomy, negative thoughts of powerlessness, failure and despair. Chronic stress can leave us vulnerable to negative suggestion, so try to focus on positives:

- Focus on your strengths
- What can you learn from this stressful circumstance ?
- Look for opportunities in the stressful situation
- What positive changes can you make ?

Change Your Behaviours

Be assertive: Being assertive means taking control and advancing your own needs and aspirations whilst remaining aware of the wishes of others. Assertiveness helps to manage stressful situations, and will in time help to reduce their frequency. Lack of assertiveness is often a function of low self-esteem and low self-confidence, factors that aggravate stress levels and can turn even relatively benign situations and events into potential crises.

The key to assertiveness is verbal and non-verbal communication. People who cannot adequately communicate their needs or wishes will create various problems for themselves. For example, the person who cannot say 'no' to others' requests is likely to be overwhelmed by external demands; the person who finds it difficult to express personal feelings and thoughts will lack self-fulfillment and not be comfortable with his or her own identity, an overly aggressive style of communication will prevent an individual from forming close personal relationships.

We all display different degrees of passive, aggressive or assertive behaviour, at different times and in different situations. Problems arise when a particular response is not in alignment for a particular situation, and we find it difficult to change to a more appropriate style of response. Improving assertiveness is about learning how to extend the range of our communication style to allow a greater flexibility of responses in different situations. It is important to acknowledge that we are all equal and have the same basic rights. Being too passive means denying one's rights by failing to express honest feelings, thoughts and beliefs, and allowing others to violate oneself. A passive person may express thoughts and feelings in such an apologetic, self-effacing manner that others can easily disregard them.

Being non-assertive means allowing people to walk all over you, denying the validity of your own needs, and surrendering control over a situation to others. This leads to stressful feelings of anxiety, powerlessness, frustration and anger.

Being assertive involves standing up for your personal rights and expressing your thoughts, feelings and beliefs directly, honestly and spontaneously in ways that don't infringe the rights of others. Assertive people respect themselves and others, and take responsibility for their actions and choices. They recognize their needs and ask openly and directly for what they want. If they fail in these efforts, for whatever reason, they may feel disappointed, but their self-confidence remains intact. They are not reliant on the approval of others.

Useful verbal and non-verbal assertive skills include the ability to:

- Establish good eye contact, but do not stare.

- Stand or sit comfortably without fidgeting.

- Talk in a firm steady voice instead of rambling or shouting.

- Use gesture to emphasize points (hands, facial expressions, body posture).

- Use statements such as 'I think', 'I feel'.

- Use empathetic statements of interest such as 'What do you think', 'How do you feel?'.

- Be concise and to the point. State clearly the message you want the other person to hear.

The more you stand up for yourself the higher your self-esteem. Your chances of getting what you want out of life improve greatly when you let others know what you want and stand up for your own rights and needs. Expressing negative feelings at the appropriate time avoids the build-up of resentment. Being less self-conscious and anxious, and less driven by the need for self-protection and control, you will be able to manage stress more successfully, and to love and appreciate yourself and others more easily.

Assert your rights:

1. I have the right to express my feelings.
2. I have the right to express my opinions and beliefs.
3. I have the right to say 'yes' and 'no' for myself.
4. I have the right to change my mind.
5. I have the right to say 'I don't understand'.
6. I have the right simply to be myself, and not act for the benefit of others.
7. I have the right to decline responsibility for others' problems.
8. I have the right to make reasonable requests of others.
9. I have the right to set my own priorities.
10. I have the right to be listened to, and taken seriously.

Get Organised

Being chronically disorganized, either at work or in the home, is one of the most common causes of stress.

Stressful environments are minimized when you impose a system or a form of structure: this offers security against unexpected problems from arising.

Too inflexible a pattern would be impractical, but keeping a diary, writing lists and prioritizing duties all help to prevent stressful situations. Writing down objectives, duties and activities helps to make them seem more tangible and surmountable.

Don't try to overload your mind with too much information. If you are already stressed there is more chance of you forgetting vital references and data. If you keep control over what you are doing there is less chance of escalating into professional and personal chaos.

Sharing Your Problems

As an old saying goes 'a problem shared is a problem halved'. People who keep things to themselves carry a considerable and unnecessary burden. Talking through a problem with others can be the first step to eliminating it. It is worth developing a support system made up of a few trusted relatives, colleagues or friends to talk to when you are upset or worried. Often it's not events themselves that are stressful but how we perceive them. Another form of communication that may be helpful is writing, for example in a private journal at home, or even letters to oneself, which should then be destroyed. The value is in expressing the feelings and getting them out. Rereading the letter just reinforces the upset and reawakens the anger.

Humour

Humour is a wonderful stress-reducer and antidote to unpleasant upsets, both at home and at work; we often laugh hardest when we have been feeling most tense. Laughter relieves muscular tension, improves breathing, regulates the heart beat and pumps endorphins, the body's natural painkillers into the bloodstream. If you feel adventurous you may seek out a form of yoga which incorporates laughing into the session. It is called 'Laughing Yoga', schools have been set up all over the world. If you can't access one then you could invest in a DVD program and do it the comfort of your own home.

Diversion and Distraction

Take time out, it could be anything from a short walk to a holiday, to get away from the things that are bothering you. This will obviously not resolve the problem, but it gives you a break and a chance for your stress levels to decrease. Then, you can return to deal with issues feeling more rested and in a better frame of mind.

Various Therapies for Stress

- **Have more fun:** Do things that you enjoy and that help you to relax.

- **Express your feelings:** Emotions need regular venting, and unexpressed emotions are the building blocks of stress, pain, and illness.

- **Get good sleep:** Poor sleep or sleep habits do not let your body really rest, discharge tensions, and recharge.

- **Learn relaxation exercises**. E.g. Yoga or Tai Chi or breathing exercises.

- **Exercise:** Regular physical exercise is one of the best ways to clear your tensions and feel good, with more energy and a better attitude toward life.

- **Develop good relationships:** It is important to have friends in whom you can confide and find support. Those who love and accept you and will advise but not judge you are your true friends. It is also very meaningful to be a true friend to another.

- **Experience love and satisfying sex:** A primary relationship that is loving, sensual, and sexual can also be a major stress reducer. However, if you do not have this in your life, there are many other therapies that are helpful. Often, an intense relationship can also be a stressor. It is important to find a relative balance in all that you do and in your life as a whole.

- **Change perceptions and attitudes:** When ideas or views are not serving you, it is wise to examine and adapt them. It is important to learn to respond to life's situations and not react as intensely.

Herbs and Supplements Helpful For Stress
Chamomile, Horsetail, Siberian Ginseng, Spirulina, Vitamin C, Valerian root, Maca root.

Tasks for This Week:

1. Note which areas of your life had a low score on the Life Analysis Chart.

2. Pay attention and take some action to improve the low score areas.

3. Make small achievable goals – like "I will start walking 15 minutes a day" or "I will spend more quality time with my child".

4. Choose a stress-reducing activity to incorporate in your life.

5. Assert your rights

11 WEEK ELEVEN

Wearing Your Party Hat !

Today was good. Today was fun. Tomorrow is another one. - Dr. Seuss

Play

Quite simply ….. take time out and have Some Fun !

Life's door, love's door, God's door – they all open when you are playful. They all become closed when you become serious. – Osho

Taking Time Out for Ourselves

Most of us experience some guilt when taking the time for ourselves. We continue to repeat negative and energy draining messages to ourselves, such as, "You're wasting time !" or "I should be spending time with the kids," or "You should be doing something more productive."

They have come to us from parents, teachers or others, and are often hard to turn off.

If you still need justification to allow yourself to play, then try this one:

Pampering and spoiling yourself is the best preventative medicine currently available !

Just Play. Have Fun. Enjoy The Game. - Michael Jordan.

We all need to be good to ourselves. Health and wellbeing includes this balancing of challenge and nurturance. When we are loved and cared for, almost anything is easy. When we are deprived, tired, needy, even the smallest detail becomes an enormous task. The alternatives and possibilities for nourishment are limited only by our old habits, by our fear of trying the untried. Nourishing yourself is well worth the risk involved.

Write a list "What nourishes me.... ". Some examples are:
- Long periods of silence
- Walks along the beach or in nature
- Dancing
- Spending quality time with my children
- Listening to your favourite music
- Hobby
- Classical music
- Pets

Seriousness

"The weight of the burden is the seriousness with which we take our separate and individual selves. – Thomas Merton"

Achieving your health and wellness goals is serious stuff or so we have been led to believe. You just have to take a look at some of the books that deal with the subject. What you frequently find are predictions of dire consequences if you fail to follow certain methods.

"Experts" demonize specific foods, or give horror stories about the lack of vitamins, or what traditional techniques can do to you, along with lists of do's and don'ts, and diets, and warnings about the cancer-causing qualities of almost everything. It's enough to drive anyone crazy !

And the subject of health is not the only one to be taken "seriously ". The same attitudes and beliefs permeate our approaches to religion, family affairs, politics ..... everybody is giving us the same message "You've really got to start taking this more seriously!"…and we do…

Seriousness creates anxiety and tension.

Seriousness creates judgment. It demands that we assign meaning to mystery, that we leave no question unanswered, that we catalogue, evaluate, and institutionalize every aspect of our lives.

Seriousness is actually an aspect of overblown self-importance, as Thomas Merton mentions above.
When we can't laugh at ourselves, it is because we are guarding our defenses, trying to be right, or good, or healthy.

Trying to keep to some schedule that can't ever be broken is stressful and can be a form of self-obsession at its best. When every little thing about ourselves and our world is assigned some super-critical importance, we have lost perspective.

We've placed ourselves, "me" at the center of the universe, and are determined that nothing must move us from our place.

Whatever breaks our excessive seriousness leads us to play and to the revitalization that play brings. Keeping that in mind, you may want to try out some of the following exercises for breaking seriousness.

Exercises for Breaking Seriousness

"Lighten up":   Choose a good-natured phrase that you can say to yourself often as a reminder to stop being so serious. "Give me a break" "Snap out of it ....." "Doing the best I can ..."

Mirror, Mirror: For some people the simple act of looking in the mirror and making funny faces is enough to break a serious mood.

Screaming in the Car: With your car safely parked, roll up the windows and scream, rant, and rave at the top of your lungs.

Dance till You Drop: Put on the wildest music you can find. Dance until you exhaust your seriousness (this is also wonderful for weight control and breathing).

Singin' the blues: For a brief period, exaggerate your mood, or your fears, to the point of absurdity. Sing them in a blues tune. Act out the most pitiful, burdened, suffering creature you can become. Give yourself a name. Be ridiculous. Start laughing as soon as possible.

Healing Laughter

Therapeutic humor is any intervention that promotes health and wellness by stimulating a playful discovery, expression, or appreciation of the absurdity or incongruity of life's situations. This intervention may enhance health or be used as a complementary treatment of illness to facilitate healing or coping, whether physical, emotional, cognitive, social, or spiritual.
– The American Association of Therapeutic Humor.

Raymond Moody Jr., M.D. has used laughter and humour with his patients for many years. He claims laughter helps to take your mind off pain and problems and catalyzes the basic will to live.

Critics of this "mind over matter" approach credit the placebo effect for its positive outcome. If you believe something strongly enough you will produce it.

Then all we have to do is learn the skills for fostering such a belief. As we begin to understand the secrets of the brain, we learn that our thoughts do trigger the pituitary gland, which directs the rest of the endocrine system. The role that these glands play in establishing the body's equilibrium has been known for centuries.
Now that we have gained some insight into how it all happens….let's keep laughing !

Tasks for This Week:

1. Take some time out for yourself everyday – even if it is just 15 minutes.

2. When you catch yourself becoming too serious… practice one of the Breaking Seriousness exercises.

3. Start a hobby if you do not already have one. Have fun ! It could be dancing lessons, rock climbing, painting, quilting, fishing, etc…

4. Laugh ! Laugh ! And Laugh !

12 WEEK TWELVE

Conscious Living

The Problems with Our Current Health Care Mentality

We have asked our medical professionals to take care of us, to be responsible for our lives.

"Doctor, doctor, please put me back together again ! ASAP !"

Experts are necessary in all aspects of life. The problem is not that we use experts. The problem is that we often shift *all* responsibility to someone or something outside ourselves.

To take charge of your own life and health implies taking calculated risks.

It means recognizing that you have choices, and it carries with it your willingness to live with the consequences of those choices.

Self-Responsibility = Self-Trust

There are no absolute answers when it comes to the subject of health. "What should I eat? How long should I exercise ? Which supplements are most beneficial ? What form of treatment is best ?"

You must learn to balance what you know and what the "experts" tell you. If you create your life about self-responsibility and love, then the burden can be transformed into an opportunity, and the questions can become the force to propel you for learning, experimenting, trusting and loving this brilliant and paradoxical creation – yourself .

Love Means

- Honouring your uniqueness, respecting and enjoying the uniqueness of others.

- Listening to your own heart and treasuring your own inner wisdom.

- Responding to life's challenges as opportunities for growth, rather than as problems.

- Caring for all aspects of yourself – body, mind, emotions, spirit – and sharing your caring with others.

- Exercising compassion for your weaknesses, and forgiving yourself and others.

- Experiencing yourself as your own best friend, and remaining faithful to yourself, especially during the down and out rough and tough times.

- Realising that you are connected with all things and acting in a congruent way aligned with that awareness.

- Being truthful with yourself and others.

- Celebrating the irrepressible process of life.

Loving yourself is what it's all about…

As you fall in love with yourself, you naturally get healthier and feel more vibrant.
When you love yourself you automatically love your body, your emotions, your intelligence, your spiritual nature.

It is to trust, accept, understand, and forgive yourself. Love is not out there waiting to be found; it is within you, wanting to be recognised.

Forgiving Yourself and Others

The willingness to accept things as they are is the first step towards lasting change. Without the compulsiveness of "have to's", changing can be a pleasant and thrilling adventure.

Resignation leads to ➔ *acceptance* ➔ *forgiveness*

Acceptance leads to compassion and forgiveness. You cannot force yourself to forgive yourself or others. Any life change, positive or negative, entails some grief, some letting go of what was.

Grieving takes time; acceptance and forgiveness are generally the results of adequate grieving.

To forgive means to be willing to refuse to hold onto the past; to release grievances; possibly even to reconcile, although this won't always be possible when another person is involved. As long as you are at peace with a certain situation then that is what counts.

Forgiveness of yourself or others often brings with it a relaxation in the body and a peace of mind. This harmony is the essence of health and the heart of wellbeing.

Guilt Vs Regret

It's important not to confuse guilt with regret.

Guilt results from doing something that we knew was "wrong" at the time.

Regret comes from later learning that we could have done something better.

When we understand the difference between guilt and regret, we can move beyond blaming ourselves for what we didn't know or weren't able to do at the time.

Even when we have the correct information, sometimes cultural and economic conditions limit our ability to implement what we know would be the best decision to make or the best course of action to take.

Loving Planet Earth !

It is important to recognize that our daily individual choices affect our planet's wellness.

It is a well known fact that about 20% of the world's population uses 80% of the world's resources. This is rather wasteful !

"Think globally, Act locally !" – Anonymous !

One vote does make a difference. The more responsible and aware we become in our own lives, the more we will see and enjoy our interdependence with one another.

"We're sitting on our blessed Mother Earth from which we get our strength and determination, love and humility - all the beautiful attributes that we've been given. So turn to one another; love one another; respect one another; respect Mother Earth; respect the waters - because that's life itself!" Phil Lane Snr

Living Lightly

"Living lightly on the planet" is an expression used by people who are conscious of their "energy footprint" and are attempting to minimize it.

Live simply so that others may simply live. - Mohandas K. Gandhi

Americans, on average, require twenty-six acres (10.5 hectares) of land per person to support their lifestyle, compared, to a worldwide average of seven acres.

Developing nations average three to five acres.
People who live lightly on the earth consciously evaluate their behaviors with regard to how they may enhance or disrupt the natural balance of all things. Your health and wellbeing and that of our children depend on this.
This may be from the exhaust fumes from cars, the chlorofluorocarbons destroying the planet's ozone layer, the urban sprawl eliminating our green space, herbicides and pesticides poisoning our soil and consequently our food.

Mankind's irrational destruction of nature bothers me a lot. Mankind is slowly committing suicide, or not so slowly. Each day it accelerates, producing all kinds of wastes—corporal, industrial, atomic—poisoning the earth, the sea and the air. He destroys the very environment that gives him sustenance. Centuries and centuries of civilization to arrive at this? What a piece of work is man! No other animal would be so stupid. Plagues of locusts are sporadic, they have a limit..." - Luis Bunuel, 1977

Thinking About Growing Your Own ?

Growing your own food can be a very pleasurable and satisfying experience. Not only will you have tastier fruits and vegetables, you'll save money and get a little exercise and sunshine at the same time.
An added benefit is that you can eliminate or control the chemicals used such as the fertilizers, pesticides, and herbicides.

Feeding Our Planet

About 25,000 people die every day of hunger or hunger-related causes, while we pursue the luxury of deciding between chicken or fish, health food or junk food, high protein or carbohydrates.

The reasons given for mass malnutrition range from the simplistic and insensitive to the frightening and complex:

- It's nature's way of population control.
- People are lazy and ignorant.

- The rich will demand what they have come to enjoy.
- We have upset the ecological balance.
- Food costs have risen with the rising costs of oil.
- Food corporations control the world.

And the situation continues to worsen… Any decision for high-level wellness as a way of life must take this reality into account.

The choices we make will impact all the people who share our planet. They affect the conditions of our soil, the prices we have to pay for food, and its availability to others.

This means that we ought to become more responsible and act on the following:

- Become informed.
- Resist waste and greed…. REDUCE, REUSE, RECYCLE !
- Possibly change our diets and eating habits.
- Work for equitable distribution of food and rightful control of the land.
- Do everything within our power to end starvation.

A balanced, nutritious diet belongs to all of us.

Confronting and Accepting Our Fears

Fear is an unpleasant emotion caused by the belief that someone or something is dangerous, likely to cause pain, or a threat.

It serves as a protection by causing us to retreat and pull back into ourselves so that we may reassess the situation and accumulates a needed supply of energy for fighting or fleeing.

Fear happens when we can no longer trust something or someone, or when we anticipate the breakdown of one of our security systems. It can be a physically painful emotion because it involves contraction and constriction of the body.

People cope with their fears in a variety of ways. Some people frantically fill their homes with appliances and furniture, their closets with new clothes or shoes, their calendars with activities, or their mouths with food when what they are really searching for is a way to deal with fear.

Others withdraw into fantasy, hide behind computer screens, or build walls of books and papers to protect themselves from the world of real live people who can hurt them.

The paradox is that an immense amount of fear is created as we spend our lives trying to escape fear.
It takes courage to confront your fears. It also helps to share them with others and give yourself lots of positive acknowledgement for each bit of progress that you have accomplished.

Keep in mind, however, that the point is not to eliminate fear which is a natural human response.

The point is to recognise it and befriend it. People who accomplish great things are those who move forward with their fears, not because they have no fear.

Anger Expression

Anger is the emotional response to what we see as an injustice or frustration. It is a powerful emotion which cannot be ignored thinking that it will go away.

If repressing your anger is a habitual response then you are likely to get into trouble.

For example, constantly grinding or tensing your jaw can misalign the dental bite, induce headaches, destroy teeth, and detract a person's physical appearance.

Unexpressed anger can feed resentment and lead to unpredictable explosions that upset your relationships and your mental balance.

It is OK to feel angry. It is OK to express it in ways that will not hurt others or yourself. ….

Punching pillows or a boxing bag helps to get some of the emotion out of your system.

Ask yourself. "What am I really angry about ?" "Why does it make me feel sad or scared ?"

Share the fact that you are feeling angry – or sad, or afraid – with the person or persons involved, and let them know how you see the situation.

Remember to take the other person's feelings into account.

Be effective, rather than right. It helps to realize that whether you are right or wrong is not the real issue in working through a "feeling" situation.

The real issue is; will the problem be effectively dealt with ? As to who is really at fault, that's a waste of time. To solve the problem effectively, it may be required that you drop self-righteousness and aim at understanding the other.

Decide what you are going to do. After the other person has shared their feelings, and you've each had a chance to see the situation from another perspective, you're in an ideal place to apply your best problem-solving skills to the situation.

Strive for a win-win solution, one that allows both or all involved to maintain dignity and self-respect while getting their needs met as much as possible.

Not all problems or people are easily dealt with, nor will every sharing session have a happy ending. Be patient with yourself and others.

Saying No without Feeling Guilty

Although guilt is not one of the primary feelings (anger, fear, sadness, and joy are), it is so pervasive in our culture that it needs some primary treatment. Guilt is a mixture of both fear and anger and acts like an internal smoke screen.

It allows us to feel bad about something but prevents us from seeing alternatives and doing anything effective to change the situation.

Guilt is widespread among those who have been trained from a very young age to "not feel OK" about themselves. Guilt usually covers up anger about the "should" they have swallowed that can never be properly digested with all the demanding and disapproving parental voices both within and without that can never be silenced.

Those who are preoccupied with guilt miss the opportunity to constructively channel their emotion into actually alleviating or solving the problem.

It is much more comfortable to keep one's familiar misery and perpetuate the cycle of self-depreciation than it is to risk the unknowns that come with being empowered and content.

Learning to say no and stand one's ground rather than excessively giving in to others, is a good starting point in breaking guilt patterns.

Experiencing and Expressing Joy

You experience joy when you realize some gain: it could be anything from finding a money note on a pavement, to receiving a compliment, to understanding and supporting the people that you love.

Joy can be sabotaged when we mistrust having too much of a good thing. We often find ourselves expecting the worst so we won't be disappointed.

Some place deep inside, many of us are afraid to open up to joy because we are afraid of losing it. Sooner or later, we think, it's got to end.

The result of this closing down can be emotional dullness, a gray world, a guarded heart, and a lonely existence even in the midst of abundance.

If only we open up our senses … joy can be found everywhere – in looking at a flower, breathing sea air, touching a leaf, gazing at a magnificent sunset.

Yet many of us miss these moments, and the possibility of joy, because we are too busy, too tired, too "mature", or too bored.

One of the magical benefits of setting our sights on health and wellness is an opening to this richness – a heightened sense of joy in all aspects of our lives.

 We may naturally feel joyful as a result of some spontaneous occurrence or it may evolve gradually as a consequence of our choices, activities, or behaviours such as these:

- Recognizing a problem (fatigue, overweight, etc...)
- Deciding to confront a problem
- Following an early morning jogging or swimming program
- Feeling a sense of wellbeing or joy

One of the best disease-preventative and healing strategies that we know is the infusion of joy with the mind and body.

Attracting Positive or Negative Attention

When someone gives us attention, it generally provides a form of stimulation or recognition.

Positive attention may come to us in the form of hugs, smiles or loving words. Negative attention as cold stares, reprimands or brush offs.

Whenever people acknowledge you in any way, in a positive or negative manner, perhaps with applause or maybe with censure you are affected and "touched" in one form or another.

To be noticed in these ways is to be acknowledged and realized that we exist. It is this realization which is absolutely essential for survival.

Our need for receiving positive attention is inextricably linked with our general state of health.
In his work with cancer patients, Carl Simonton M.D. observed:

"The biggest single factor that I can find as a predisposing factor to the actual development of cancer is the loss of a serious love object, occurring six to eighteen months prior to the onset of the disease."

The love object is frequently a child or spouse which is a primary source of attention. When that is lost, it can lead to destructive means of compensation. Nobody wants cancer or another serious disease, but everyone wants attention !

Sometimes a problem develops because we have collected a poisonous supply of negative attention. Many of us tend to store it up until it eats away at us from within.

Hurts, anger, fear, deep sadness. These all create an energy which will look for an outlet somewhere in the body if it doesn't get conscious recognition or expression.

Such outlets include:

- Smoking or overeating
- Driving recklessly
- Gritting Teeth
- "Getting" a sore throat, an asthmatic attack or a headache.
- An extra rush of adrenaline into the blood stream that makes us feel wired.
- A stress-related condition such as constipation, a skin disorder, eye fatigue, or an ulcer
- Building defenses, by withdrawal and depression, to keep us from being hurt again.

When we don't understand our real needs or how to fulfill them, we are left with a void that is all too easily filled by illness or dangerous habits.

As children, many of us got some of our most nurturing attention when we were sick.

Some of us still use the same tactics as adults.
We think we have to break down totally before we can get the help and attention we need.

While it would be simplistic to assume that serious illness is the result of one factor alone, many health conditions are significantly improved when friendship, attention, and a support system are added to treatment or healing methods.

Attention heals !

Close Friends

It is important to have several close friends with whom you can talk about anything and who will support you in being the best possible person you can be.
It is important to keep in mind that support does **NOT EXCLUDE** negative feedback or even criticism from others.

It is a mark of greatness to be able to face the truth and be willing to hear it, no matter how clumsily it is expressed or how painful it may feel.

It is possible, especially among caring friends, to move beyond the realm of winning and losing, being wrong or being right.

Life is tough anyway. Alone, it may appear to be intolerable.

Remember that it is absolutely necessary to ask for and be open to help, just as it is essential to ask for and be open to love.

A twenty-year survey of adults in the United States reported that, regardless of health problems, people who participated in formal social networks of some type outlived those who did not.

An affiliation with a social network was found to be the strongest predictor of longevity, even above age, sex, or health.

When people are counting on you, you have a reason to get up in the morning.

Expressing Love, Warmth and Concern

Studies have clearly shown that people who can experience and express their love and concern live longer, healthier lives.

Being able to express our feelings of love doesn't just cause us to feel better – the other person gains a sense of well being as well.

What more powerful form of attention could you get than to have someone you care about say " I love you"? And what greater impact could you have on your world than to give your love freely, without reservation, without fear ?

Unfortunately, few of us dare to open up enough to give or receive love.

Typically, we tie up much life energy in restricting the flow of love because we are afraid – we fear rejection, fear strong emotions being aroused, fear intimacy, or fear vulnerability.

Like the ground we walk on, love supports us in all we do. Blocking love, whether it is self-love or love for or from others, will inexorably have a negative effect on our happiness and health.

Love is not something you can analyze and define. In fact, attempting to do so is likely to keep you from being able to experience it.

Love is letting go – letting go of fears, grievances, and judgments. The secret is simply to allow it to happen.

"Love is giving people the space to be who they are, and who they are not. – Werner Erhard"

Creating Our Own Reality

We create our own reality with our every thought, word and action.

"Watch your thoughts, for they become words. Watch your words, for they become actions. Watch your actions, for they become habits. Watch your habits, for they become character. Watch your character, for it becomes your destiny."

Florence Scovel Shinn once said …"That Life is a game of boomerangs. Our thoughts, deeds and words return to us sooner or later with astounding accuracy.

Before you think, do or say anything – imagine what it would be like to receive what you are sending…

The Mind Healing the Body

We know that this is possible because of the placebo effect. The placebo effect is one of the clearest demonstrations of how thinking affects the body. Patients obtain relief even though the doctor has given them a sugar pill, an injection of saline solution or some other innocuous substance. The placebo causes emotional calming and can actually change the physical experience within the body. A negative aspect to the placebo is that it depends upon deception. The doctor knows that he is giving a harmless substance yet the patient doesn't.

Can we trigger the mind-body connection without being deceived ? Is there a way for each and every one of us to use our mind to influence his body consciously ?

To insure a stronger mind-body connection, keep the following in mind:

- The mind contributes to getting well.
- The mind doesn't contribute to getting sick.
- The body is in constant communication with the mind.
- This communication benefits both the physical and mental aspects of being well.

All four aspects are involved when the placebo effect works.

- The person's mind cooperates with the treatment and trusts it.

- The body is fully aware of this trust.

- There is open communication. As a result of this, the cells throughout the body participate in a healing response. The healing system as a whole is incredibly complex and all but impossible to explain as a whole. We only know parts of how it operates, such as our knowledge of antibodies and the immune response to infection.

Yet somehow, for all its complexity, the healing system can be triggered by a simple intention of the mind.

To be your own placebo, then, requires the same conditions that apply in a classic placebo response:

- You trust what is happening.
- You deal with doubt and fear.
- You don't send conflicting messages that get tangled with each other.
- You have opened the channels of mind-body communication.
- You let go of your intention and let the healing system do its work.

On a final note, I am not advising anyone to stop conventional medical treatment or to reject medical help. Yet it is important to have in mind that a positive mental state can help in any healing process.

The Brain – Heart Connection

Research has been conducted at the Institute of Heart Math in California on how the brain functions.

Their findings show that our perceptions, mental and emotional attitudes, immune system, and decision-making abilities are all related to the electromagnetic frequencies broadcasted by our heart.

These frequencies are many, many times stronger than brainwave frequencies and can be measured from several feet outside the body.

They influence our own brain rhythms as well as the brain rhythms of others nearby. It is through this mechanism that the heart appears to influence the brain and live up to its popular reputation of being more than just a pump.

Studies show that the heart is a powerful agent for transforming perceptions, resolving challenges, and manifesting values that benefit everyone.

Recurring feelings of frustration, worry, stress, and anger cause heart rhythms to become unbalanced and incoherent.

These feelings are detrimental not only to the physical heart but also to the brain, hormonal production, and the immune system.

Even remembering an upsetting experience can reduce the heart's pumping efficiency by 5 to 7 percent and decrease the immune system's potency for many hours.

On the other hand, forgiveness, appreciation, and love engender coherent, harmonious heart rhythms and affect the physical heart's electrical output, as seen in an ECG. These feelings generate heart frequencies that are radiated to every cell in the body and boost the immune system.

One five-minute episode of feeling genuine care or compassion enhances the immune system, causing a gradual climb in IgA (an antibody, one of the body's first defenses against colds, flu's and infections), for the next six hours.

Feelings of happiness and joy benefit the white blood cells that are needed for healing and defense against invading pathogens, including cancer and virus-infected cells.

The next time you are sick get some strong doses of nurturing and fun filled time rather than just reaching for the vitamin C !

Worrying

The biggest energy drain is worry. Worries are often closely related to a sense of guilt or shame and they typically run as strong background programs in our minds.

When you create negative mental pictures or repeat worry messages to yourself about illness, accident, failure, or weakness of any kind, it impacts your body and influences the reality you create.

Mind and body are connected, and worrying about illness wears down the body's natural defense mechanism.

Truthful and Caring Communications

Small talk may not be bad, but it is generally not all that nourishing. The failure to express our real feelings can rob us of energy.

Communicating with others is more intimate when you are able to share your true feelings, rather than merely talking about the weather or hobbies.

Feelings are not always pleasant subjects and most of us have trouble expressing negative feelings.

If the relationship is an intimate one or one that requires the building and maintenance of trust, it is all the more vital that clear, truthful, and caring communications is the foundation.

By talking with others, we share our thoughts, and thus we share ourselves. As we share ourselves, we get to learn about each other and the world around us. This then allows us to be open, to learn, and to grow.

"The advantage of telling the truth is that you don't have to remember what you said." – Mark Twain

Avoiding Absolutes, Generalizations, Labels, and Judgments

It is natural to form judgments about the world. We all have generalizations about the sexes, other age groups, and other cultures, but if we use those generalizations to stereotype, "write off", or oversimplify our ideas about another person, we miss the opportunity to know them better or to learn from them, and expand our understanding of the world we share.

Appreciate that there is some truth in generalizations, but don't make them the sum total of all your communications.

Assertive Communication

Assertiveness basically means the ability to express your thoughts and feelings in a way that clearly states your needs and keeps open the lines of communication with the one another.

By blocking our feelings, we may create tensions that collect in different parts of our bodies.

Eventually they may surface as illness of some sort. It takes a great deal of effort to continually walk the fence, trying to please all the people, all the time. But that's what we must do to remain "the nice guy" or "sweetheart".

We have to swallow hard, breathe lightly, walk on tiptoe, and maybe end up with stomach ulcers, or arthritis, or cancer. The body will allow just so much repressed emotion to collect. Then it will have its way.

Our reluctance to be assertive often stems from confusing this type of communication with aggression, but they are simply not the same.

"Shut up !" which is a hostile approach or "Please can you be quiet" is a firm but assertive approach.

Hostility breeds hostility. Firmness with respect leaves the other intact.

It is your right as a human being to be able to express an unpopular opinion, to say no when that is what you really mean, to take care of your own needs, to be in charge of your own life or to let others take control as appropriate.

To refrain from doing so in important situations may rob you of your peace of mind, your self-esteem, and your body's natural inclinations towards inner harmony and a general feeling of contentment and inner peace.

Owning Our Mistakes

It's quite stressful to worry and question what might happen if or when somebody finds out about something we've done or neglected to do.

Owning up to our mistakes, quickly, is a healthier option. In this way we can channel our energy and use it in more life-enhancing ways.

When it comes to apologizing or telling the truth about our mistakes or any other mistakes, it's crucial to make the distinction between the essential goodness of yourself, on the one hand, and your behaviours on the other.

Everybody breaks things; everybody breaks down, at times. Nobody fulfills the perfect ideal !

We are not defined by our mistakes unless we want to be. We have difficulty separating a label from the person or thing and we often take on unnecessary guilt or blame because we have identified it with our shortcomings or accidents.

Certainly this is true in our culture: because of our perceived need to be "right", assigning blame is most likely the first line of response.

This form of defensiveness may easily overshadow the more important need to solve the problem that has arisen as a result of the mistake.

Apologize if appropriate, own up to the truth as necessary, acknowledge your own essential goodness and move on.

Listening Skills

We all need to develop our active listening skills. Most of us have selective hearing and allow much of what we hear to go in one ear and out the other.

Learning to listen brings tremendous and often immediate rewards that contribute to health and happiness on all sides.

When we meet the other on common ground, we relieve stress and we provide them with caring and attention. To be listened to is to be acknowledged as a worthwhile human being – and that's the best medicine there is.

Listening.

Communication specialist Jud Morris sums up the ways in which we block or discourage understanding by poor habits of listening:

- Evaluation, judgment. We are so busy planning our attack, or criticizing the other's message, that we often do not really hear what is being said.

- Jumping to conclusions. We jump to conclusions, filling in our own details before the other has had a chance to explain himself or herself.

- "We're all the same." We assume that other people think as we do.

- Attitude, the closed mind. We tune out people with whom we don't agree.

- Lack of Attention. We let our minds wander.

- Wishful hearing. We tend to hear just what we want to hear, or expect to hear.

- Excessive Talking. We interrupt or dominate the conversation so that the other doesn't get a chance to adequately express his or her ideas.

- Unclear words. We fail to find out what the other means by the particular words he or she chooses.

- Lack of Humility. We feel that we must express our superiority by speaking or contradicting the other.

- Fear. We avoid listening with understanding because we are afraid that the other may challenge some long-held belief. We are afraid to be threatened by a new idea.

Love

Love is not something we find.
Love is something we build.
– Bhai Sahib.

Living with a Purpose

The search for meaning involves asking these basic questions. Who am I ? Why am I here ? Where am I going ? What do I want ? What is real ?

Regardless of whether these questions are conscious or unconscious, all life activity, all energy expressions, are coloured by them.

The ongoing process of addressing these questions encourages a balanced life and provides us with a focal point toward which to direct our energy.

The great and glorious masterpiece of humanity is to know how to live with a purpose. – Montaigne.

Finding meaning is probably the most personal and most challenging issue anyone can address, because it requires looking inward and self-searching, which some find a frightening prospect.

One of the books which I thoroughly enjoyed on the subject was "Man's Search for Meaning", by Victor E. Frankl. He states

"… man's search for meaning may arouse inner tension rather than inner equilibrium … such tension is an indispensable prerequisite of mental health."

"… the meaning of life differs from man to man, from day to day and from hour to hour."

"Everyone has his own specific vocation or mission in life to carry out a concrete assignment which demands fulfillment. Therein he cannot be replaced, nor can his life be repeated. Thus, everyone's task is as unique as is his specific opportunity to implement it."

"He who has a why to live for can bear with almost any how." - Nietzsche

This is a journey you must make alone… I wish you courage, strength and joy in your exploration.

Where Do Meanings Come From Anyway ?

Meanings are made up in human minds, and perpetuated by common agreement. They vary according to place and time and heritage.

Your personal meanings vary with your need, or mood, or what you ate for breakfast.

Since meaning comes from inside of you, finding meaning will be a process of going to the source… yourself.

The Examined Life

"The unexamined life is not worth living." – Socrates

In our modern, materialistic, media-saturated society, few people take the time to ponder the questions of meaning, yet doing so is crucial to creating a balanced, purposeful, and rewarding life.

Looking at our priorities and values is a much more immediate process. Values and priorities essentially show up in how we live, not in our concepts about how we wish we could live.

This may sometimes be a hard truth to face if we say that spending quality time with our children is a priority, but we continually put dozens of other tasks ahead of spending time with them, then our priorities are skewed, and our values are questionable.

While there are millions of good excuses about why we aren't getting to do the things we say we want to do, excuses don't build satisfying relationships.

Acting in line with our values and priorities creates personal integrity and gives meaning to our lives. In contemplating what is truly meaningful to them, many people discover that experiencing and expressing love are central to their fulfillment in life.

The challenge is to transform the fear that is so rampant in our culture (often expressed as anger or impatience) into love. This can be a lifelong project that propels meaning and direction into every moment of life.

Pleasure, Meaning and Eudaimonia

Most people believe that happiness equals pleasure. A life that has more positive feelings and less negative ones is a happy life.

There are two other paths to happy lives. The meaningful life and the good life, which may not have any positive emotion at all.

This common view of happiness convinces us that Meg Ryan is the paradigmatic example of being happy, smiley, cheerful, bright-eyed and lively.

Two Things Wrong with This Idea.

There are two things radically wrong with this hedonic view. The first is that smiley ebullience is highly heritable and very hard to get more of.

This trait is called "positive affectivity" and identical twins are much more likely to share it than fraternal twins. It is not very changeable, and the best you can hope for from learning skills such as "savoring" and "mindfulness" is to help you live in the upper part of your set range of positive affectivity.

The fact that it is normally distributed means that half the population is not very smiley, cheerful, and ebullient, and not likely to become so – even with carefully reading and diligently doing the exercises in Authentic Happiness.

The second problem with the Hollywood view of happiness, as pervasive as it is, is a very poor intellectual provenance.

When Aristotle spoke of the "Eudaimonia", the good life, he was not focused on the positive feelings of pleasure such as an orgasm, a back rub, and a full stomach.

Rather, he was concerned with the "pleasures" of contemplation – which do not reside in orgasmic thrills or sensations of warmth, but in a deep absorption and immersion.

During this state there is neither thought nor feeling. You are simply one with the music.

Three Paths to Happy Lives

With regards to authentic happiness, there are three very different routes:

First, the pleasant life, consisting in having as many pleasures as possible and having the skills to amplify the pleasures. This is, of course, the only true kind of happiness in the Hollywood view.

Second, the good life, which consists in knowing what your signature strengths are, then re-crafting your work, love, friendship, leisure, and parenting to use those strengths to have more flow in life.

Third, the meaningful life, which consists of using your strengths in the service of something that you believe is larger than you are.

Important New Evidence

Until recently, the idea that there are three routes to happiness, two of which do not involve any felt positive emotion at all, was merely an untested theory.
Recent unpublished research shows startling results
Pleasure doesn't add to satisfaction.

One of the studies found that both the good life and the meaningful life were related to life satisfaction: the more eudaimonia or the more meaning, the more life satisfaction.

Astonishingly, however, the amount of pleasure in life did not add to life satisfaction.

Eudaimonia predicts satisfaction. The other study found that eudaimonia pursuits were significantly correlated with life satisfaction, whereas hedonic pursuits were not.

"Happiness is the progressive realization of a worthy ideal. - Brian Tracy

Listening To Our Inner Voice

Today we are bombarded with a multitude of self-serving and superficial messages with often conflicting directions telling us how to live our lives.

It is only by looking inward, past and through the multitude of voices that surround us, and growing quiet enough within ourselves, that we can hear, with our heart, what is true for us.

We can also cultivate our ability to listen by simply taking time alone to do something that brings us closer to nature, to our own inner self, gardening, walking in the woods or on the beach, relaxing in a park, meditation, or even settling reflectively into a welcoming corner of a coffee shop.
The process of such opening to wisdom is an expression of wisdom itself.

"At the heart of each of us, whatever our imperfections, there exists a silent pulse of perfect rhythm. A complex of waveforms and resonances, which is absolutely individual and unique, and yet which connects us to everything in the Universe" – George Leonard.

Goal Setting

Before you can have any real sense of getting somewhere, you need to know the point from which you're starting, and where you want to go.

Goal setting, action, evaluation, and redirection are a set of dynamic tools that can assist you in navigating successfully toward your desired destination.

Many of us resist setting goals and taking action that will take us closer to our goals.

We often take whatever comes along in life with half-hearted resignation, making the "best" of a situation rather than risking the disappointment and frustration we may experience when our hopes and expectations are not met.

It takes courage to call into question, and to consider changing, some of our most basic behaviours and ways of thinking.

Even if we don't accomplish all the goals we initially set for ourselves, the very process of formulating goals is energizing and life-affirming.

Exercise

Take four blank sheets of paper and write on each:
Take no more than fifteen minutes to work on each sheet, beginning with the five-year projection, and moving down to the last six months.

First Sheet: "Where/ How I want My Life to Be Five Years From Today."

Second Sheet: "Where/How I Want My Life to Be Two Years from Today."

Third Sheet: "Where/How I want my Life to be Six Months from Today."

Fourth Sheet: "How I would Spend the Next Six Months of My Life If I Knew for Sure They Would Be My Last."

Read over what you have written and look for things that are repeated or strongly expressed.

Note patterns that are emerging.

As you write, listen to your internal self-talk that may be undermining the process, saying for example, "But that can never happen" or "I don't have the money (or courage or time) to do that."

Keep moving ahead despite these self-defeating messages.

Put this exercise aside for at least a day, and do it again the next day or the next week.

Compare and contrast the results of the two experiments, and keep asking yourself, "What would I have to /do/be if I had no limitations (like time, children, money, etc.)?" So often we use our imagined limitations as defenses against clearly asserting and then setting out after what we really want.

High achievers only ask :How?" - Work to find ways to turn visions and goals into reality.

The difference between a life of greatness and a life of mediocrity is that the great move ahead with their limitations, while the mediocre stay stuck in them !!

Making Time for Your Dreams

"A dreamer is one who can only find his way by moonlight, and his punishment is that he sees the dawn before the rest of the world. - Oscar Wilde.

Most of us are so caught up in the busy-ness of life that we put off the things that are most important to us – beginning or completing that project our heart calls us to act on, or taking time with friends, children, loved ones. The pace of modern life gets faster with each passing year. Unless you take charge and resist the temptation, pressure, or expectation to keep up with it, you will likely never do the thing that you say you most want to do. Getting clear on what your goals are is the first step, but goals are meaningless unless you structure your time so you can pursue them.

Living in the Now

Looking to the future for happiness or living on past glories is a sure setup for disappointment.
Ultimately we have no assurance of anything beyond this present moment. There really is no future or past – just a continuous progression of "now" moments.

The question then is "What am I to do in the 'now' in order to experience meaning ?" Be real, live life authentically, face reality and look at what is real right now.

Taking a walk we can remind ourselves to look, smell, feel, hear what is around us.

Making love, we can remind ourselves to stay present to the body, rather than retreating into fantasy.

Life is a Mystery to Be Lived not a Problem to Be Solved !

"We stake our lives on our purposeful programs and projects, our serious jobs and endeavors. But doesn't the really important part of our lives unfold "after hours" – singing and dancing, music and painting, prayer and lovemaking, or just fooling around?"– Father William McNamara

Relax, laugh and play when things get too serious and you realize that you'll never be finished with learning, changing, and growing.

Facing Death and Finding Meaning

The culture in which we live has emphasized the prolonging of life – often supporting its quantity above its quality.

Doctors are committed to keeping us alive – as an inherent value. Consequently when death occurs it means failure. It's that simple.

But death is not the ultimate enemy, the terminal disease to wage war against, to be eliminated at all costs.

We delude ourselves in believing that medical research will discover a cure for death.

It's true that people who watch their diets, exercise, and enjoy satisfying relationships often live longer.

Nevertheless, we are all terminal, and death is our natural heritage.

"I have been able to function as a catalyst, trying to bring to our awareness that we can only truly live and enjoy and appreciate life if we realize at all times that we are finite. Needless to say I have learned these lessons from my dying patients – who in their suffering and dying realized that we have only NOW – "so have it fully and find what turns you on, because no one can do this for you!" – Elizabeth Kubler Ross

Beyond Our Limits

Contemporary culture is fascinated with the ability of the human organism to do what seems impossible, as shown by the popularity of Guinness World Records.

Every day someone shows us that what we previously thought were our limits are actually only the baselines, offering yet another challenge to be exceeded.

In these "X-games", moreover, we find that the mind's role is always paramount.

Limited beliefs lead to limited results, and vice versa.

Sri Chinmoy a spiritual teacher, author, and poet believes in inspiring others to transcend the limitations of the mind and therefore the body. He has written over 1,300 books, painted over 135,000 pieces of art, and mastering over 100 musical instruments, he has run 22 marathons and lifted over 7,000 pounds in order to show us that we don't aim high enough !!

"Reality is what we take to be true. What we take to be true is what we believe. What we believe is based upon our perceptions. What we perceive depends upon what we look for. What we look for depends upon what we think. What we think depends upon what we perceive. What we perceive determines what we believe. What we take to be true is our reality. "– Gary Zukav

Finding Inner Peace

The stress of living in the twenty-first century on planet Earth requires the programming of safety valves to keep us healthy and happy. From every direction we are bombarded with forces that tend to draw us away from ourselves.

The media tell us what we should like and dislike. Pressured jobs preoccupy us and can disturb our necessary sleep. Noises in the environment continually distract us from the task at hand. We can be left feeling like a battered boat on an angry sea – losing touch with what we really want, really believe, and ultimately, with whom we really are.

A daily practice of a stress-reduction technique ranging from a walk in the park, listening to calm music, painting, writing, exercising, gardening, deep breathing …. May help us to relax, and come to a serene place within ourselves.

Intuition and Wellness

"The intellect has little to do on the road to discovery. There comes a leap in consciousness, call it intuition or what you will, and the solution comes to you, and you don't know why or how" – Albert Einstein

Merriam- Webster's dictionary defines intuition as "quick and ready insight"; and the power of faculty of attaining to direct knowledge or cognition without evident rational thought and inference.

It is derived from Latin intueri, to see within. It is a way of knowing, of sensing the truth without explanations. In developing intuition we develop self-knowledge and self-appreciation. Self-appreciation allows us to develop self-trust.

Genuine self-trust (not inflated egoism) creates a greater sense of awe at the mystery of this life in which we are all engaged.

Living Life Authentically

There's a common misunderstanding among all the human beings who have ever been born on the earth that the best way to live is to try to avoid pain and just try to get comfortable. You can see this even in insects and animals and birds. All of us are the same.

A much more interesting, kind, adventurous, and joyful approach to life is to begin to develop our curiosity, not caring whether the object of our inquisitiveness is bitter or sweet.

(Pema Chodron, The Wisdom of No Escape and the Path of Loving- Kindness – Shambhala, 1991.

Tasks for This Week:

1. What actions can you take to start taking responsibility for your health and well being ?

2. Loving yourself – choose three actions which reflect loving yourself and others.

3. Forgive yourself or someone who has hurt you. Perhaps write a letter to yourself or to the person who has hurt you and express your feelings.

4. Are you angry about something ? What can you do to release it ? Ask yourself "What am I really angry about ?" "Why does it make me sad or scared?".

5. Take some time to reflect on your own lifestyle and ways in which you touch the earth, the water, the air.

6. What can you do to Reduce, Reuse and Recycle ?

7. Write your goals down.

8. What can you do to make your life more meaningful ? It could be as simple as volunteering at a dog shelter.

References

Kenton, Susannah and Leslie, The New Raw Energy, London, Vermilion, 1994

Travis, John W. M.D. and Ryan, Regina Sarah, Wellness Workbook - How To Achieve Enduring Health and Vitality, California, Celestial Arts, 2004

Haas, M.D., Elson, Staying Healthy With Nutrition, California, Celestial Arts, 1992.

Beling, M.D. Stephanie, Power Foods, New York, Harper Collins, 1998.

Costain BSc, SRD, Lyndel, Super Nutrients Handbook, London, Dorling Kindersley, 2001

Shape, Work Out, S.A. 2003.

Nutrition Delusion, Australia, 2001.

Balch, M.D., James F., Balch, CNC, Phyllis, A., Prescription For Nutritional Health, New York, Penguin, 2000.

(Story from BBC NEWS: http://news.bbc.coc.uk/go/pr/fr/-/2/hi/health/8524549.stm)

Source:
http://news.bbc.co.uk/1/hi/scotland/glasgow_and_west/793150 8.stm   also sees:
http://www.telegraph.co.uk/health/healthnews/4957365/Takin g-naps-increases-diabetes-risk.html

ABOUT THE AUTHOR

Barbara Karafokas was born and brought up in Zambia and now lives on the beautiful Mediterranean island of Cyprus.

She has recently become a passionate tri-athlete, is a qualified Holistic Nutritionist MSc., a Health and Wellness Expert and counsels athletes and sporty folk in sports nutrition.

Barbara brings a blend of skills to her practice and teaching. For over fifteen years she has been committed to creating awareness about the hidden dangers to health. She promotes healthy eating, a healthy lifestyle combined with an authentic Mediterranean diet, the raw food diet, wholefood supplements, herbs, exercise, meditation, stress management advice and other healthy lifestyle tips.

As a nutrition, health and wellness consultant she offers on and offline counseling. Her passion is to inspire and empower others to create the life that they dream of, free from disease.

Barbara is also the author of 'The Med Life Diet' a beginner's guide to creating healthy eating and healthy lifestyle habits & attitudes for life !

Follow The Med Life Diet on Facebook:
(https://www.facebook.com/TheMedLifeDiet)
For more information please visit:
(www.barbarakarafokas.com)

Barbara also teaches workshops based on The Med Life Diet; for availability or if you want to connect with Barbara simply send an e-mail to barbara@barbarakarafokas.com and she will get back to you within the day.

www.ingramcontent.com/pod-product-compliance
Lightning Source LLC
Chambersburg PA
CBHW061354280526
45784CB00001B/250